The
Observable
Universe

An Investigation

HEATHER
McCALDEN

HOGARTH

New York

Published in the United States by Hogarth, an imprint of Random House,
a division of Penguin Random House LLC, New York.

HOGARTH is a trademark of the Random House Group Limited, and the
H colophon is a trademark of Penguin Random House LLC.

Published in Great Britain by Fitzcarraldo Editions, London.

LIBRARY OF CONGRESS CATALOGING-IN-PUBLICATION DATA
Names: McCalden, Heather, author.
Title: The observable universe / by Heather McCalden.
Description: New York : Hogarth, [2024]
Identifiers: LCCN 2023034181 (print) | LCCN 2023034182 (ebook) |
ISBN 9780593596470 (hardcover) | ISBN 9780593596494 (ebook)
Subjects: LCSH: McCalden, Heather. | HIV infections—United States—History. |
AIDS (Disease)—United States—History. | Internet—History.
Classification: LCC RA643.83 .M35 2024 (print) | LCC RA643.83 (ebook) |
DDC 362.19697/9200973—dc23/eng/20231207
LC record available at https://lccn.loc.gov/2023034181
LC ebook record available at https://lccn.loc.gov/2023034182

Printed in the United States of America on acid-free paper

randomhousebooks.com

2   4   6   8   9   7   5   3   1

First U.S. Edition

Book design by Sara Bereta

Dead men are heavier than broken hearts.
—RAYMOND CHANDLER, *The Big Sleep*

Metaphor is halfway between the unintelligible and
the commonplace.
—ARISTOTLE, at least according to the internet

The
Observable
Universe

DIRECTIONS FOR HOW TO READ

This book is an album about grief. Every fragment is like a track on a record, a picture in a yearbook; they build on top of one another until, at the end, they form an experience.

WEIGHTLESSNESS

The precondition for all things that exist in albums is weightlessness. Images and songs have zero mass, stamps are mostly surface area, and autographs seep into their surfaces, becoming indistinguishable from them. The function of albums, long before the advent of photography or recorded sound, was to secure the particles of everyday life that might otherwise slip under the radar if not captured and pinned down: letters, old receipts, birth announcements, cookie fortunes, postcards, hair, pressed daffodils, and movie ticket stubs are items that might evaporate if not carved out of space and glued into a new chronology; albums impose themselves on their contents. There is always a beginning, middle, and end, a first place and a last place, and so the eventual arrangement of information might say more than any one object on its own.

SEASHELL HEAD

I covered one ear with one hand, and my forehead with the other, and gently twisted my face down into my clavicles, folding into a seashell. The bartender asked what I was doing.

"Hiding," I said.

"You haven't even had a drink yet."

This wasn't true exactly. I hadn't had a drink in this bar yet, but I had five beers at the art opening and a shot of gin, beforehand, to get me there.

"Who are you hiding from?"

"Ghosts."

The bartender then extracted his body from the space he was occupying and slunk down the bar, somehow leaving the impression of his outline hanging in the air in front of me as a sort of decoy. From his new location he then proceeded to slide—on a single fingertip—a menu in my direction, as if I might be leaking something. "I'm going to leave you alone now," he said, "with all that," swirling his hand in a loose figure of eight to suggest a host of specters around me.

"They're not contagious," I said, but maybe what I should have said was "I'm not contagious," except before I had time to correct myself he was gone, flirting with someone else.

I didn't normally run my mouth like this to strangers, or anyone really, but the exhibition had left me with a horrible vacant feeling. It featured a series of black-and-white portraits of naked men. They were taken with a pinhole camera the artist had placed in her vagina. The less said about this, the better.

When the bartender returned, I ordered a double shot of Basil

Hayden with a single ice cube. I theatrically raised my drink toward him in a toast, at which point it finally dawned on him I was three sheets to the wind. I wasn't just some loon who had accidentally wandered in from the street, but a person genuinely trying to wind the night down, after being stuck to a wall somewhere else. He clinked an imaginary glass against my own and then left me to my thoughts, which were black.

The bar was heaving with bodies jutting out at every conceivable angle and voices cascading in thick, jagged murmurs. Despite the noise I somehow caught a piece of a story being told in the crowd behind me. A woman suffering from intense, undiagnosed leg pain visited a temple in Cambodia for a possible cure. "A monk there told me that my heart was too heavy for my legs to support," she said, "so he walked me over to a tree and pointed. 'Leave it here!' he said. 'Bury your heart under the roots. When you go home it will not be inside you anymore, and after some time, you will forget where you left it.'"

I chugged the rest of my drink, threw on my coat, and shoved my way onto the street.

Outside, the London air stung my face and I clung to that bitter sensation until I lost track of everything else. It was late, I was shivering, and drifting like a piece of seaweed through town. The story of the woman and her legs swam in and out of my mind, and I wondered about putting my own heart into the ground when I looked at my feet and noticed they were no longer moving. It was unclear to me how long I had been stationary, but when I came to I was standing in front of a decrepit phone booth thrown off its axis by a car accident. The red exterior was severely dented and covered in a rich film of dirt. When I opened the door the inside was full of dried leaves, wadded-up McDonald's bags, crisp packets, and cigarette butts. Ads for phone sex hotlines peppered every available surface. The booth seemed to have most recently been used as a urinal, but I walked into it anyway and closed the door behind me, the bronzed faces of Crystal, Violet, Alana, Tiffany, Tiffani, and Amber Rose staring at me from ceiling to floor. In slow motion, I picked up the receiver and held it a few centimeters away from my ear. I could barely make out a dial tone. It was faint, but it was there. It sounded like a song.

LA MARATHON PHOTO

My mother, Vivian, ran the LA Marathon sometime between the late seventies and early eighties. The only evidence I have of this is a photograph in a coffee-table book celebrating the Los Angeles bicentennial.

The dust jacket, glossy and jet-black, shows the city skyline piercing the night sky. Inside, postcard-worthy images of Angeleno city life, of Olvera Street and the Hollywood Bowl, interrupt thick passages of text glorifying urban planning and architectural feats. At the dead center of the book is the marathon photo. It features a sea of tanned runners, fit and glistening in tangerine light. They wear headbands, wristbands, and tank tops with piping in primary colors. Their numbers billow across their chests like sails pulling them forward to the finish line. Near the center of all that color and motion is Vivian flashing her megawatt grin directly at the camera. The other faces, absorbed in purpose, look forward or down at their feet, and some blur, appearing in frame only as streaks of motion.

NETWORK

Several links form a network, like a tethered bank of office computers hissing and pulsing with electrical static; the computers are joined, "linked," but are also tied into a configuration, into a relationship, with one another. "Link" is a verb and a noun—an action and a situation.

We might ask how information travels in such a situation. It flows. Like blood. It circulates down veins and chambers. It spreads.

LOS ANGELES REFRACTION

Running underneath Los Angeles are several currents of myth. They propel the city forward with the same force as the material ones of traffic and population density. Their motion generates a field of visual distortion and all the images ever taken of the city rise out of the concrete like heat waves and bleed over rooftop pools and stucco houses, Bel Air mansions and strip mall parking lots, taco trucks and palm fronds, canyon roads and chainlink fences, and the consequent haze disorients. It both enthralls and repulses, confusing traditional navigational strategies. Tourists get nervous as hell when they can't locate the geographic center of town. It means they can't traverse it in any normative sense, and so the landscape fails to assemble itself in any familiar manner. Los Angeles is then written off as "weird," "nightmarish," and "impossible," and while it is all of those things, it is also a place where anything can happen. Most things, in fact, have.

ORGANIC MATTER

When a person you love dies from organic matter and not from a car crash or a gunshot wound, the matter goes straight into you because: *it* continues to survive. Your loss creates a vacuum and the organic matter—say, a virus—rushes in to fill it. It exists there then, underneath your sternum, below the cartilage, mutating, evolving, spreading, as if it were a living thing, so you let it invade your nervous system, your organs, and just like that it becomes part of you, part of your story—a virus after all is made up of letters, just like words, and it serves as an unbroken transmission broadcast through time saying: I go on. I go on. I go on—

OLDEST KNOWN SPECIMEN

In 1959, a blood sample is taken from a man in Léopoldville, the capital of the Belgian Congo. Thirty-nine years later, during a global search for the origin of HIV, the sample will test positive for the virus. To this day, it remains the oldest known specimen of HIV in the world.

TO HOLD TO

"Observe," according to the Online Etymology Dictionary, originates from "late 14c., *observen*," which means "to hold to (a manner of life or course of conduct), carry out the dictates of, attend to in practice, to keep, follow." This suggests that what we calibrate our minds to creates a bond, a physical connection to the thing observed: a holding. Observing religious ceremonies, holidays, tax laws, anniversaries, solstices, weather patterns, reservation times, and shopping mall hours forms points of contact between the self and external phenomena. By extension, it follows that the whole world might be collected through a series of links—

JAPANESE PHONE BOOTH

I heard a story on National Public Radio about a telephone booth in Ōtsuchi, Japan. A man in his seventies built it, painted it white, and placed it on a hill in his garden where it overlooked the sea. The interior of the booth held a black rotary phone, a pad of paper, and a pen.

The man, who had been a gardener, began building the booth after his cousin passed away in 2010. The two had been close, and there were many things left unsaid. In interviews the man explains the idea for the project came to him because his "thoughts couldn't be relayed over a regular phone line," so he created a poetic cord of transmission, a direct connection to the ether, where words and sentences could diffuse into the atmosphere.

The booth was completed shortly after the 2011 tsunami, and then people just started showing up to use it. They used it to call the afterlife. They used it to call their missing parts. They called landlines and mobile phones. They twisted digits into the rotary and then paused, listening to phantom rings before speaking.

The radio segment played recordings of these conversations. The clips ranged from casual updates, grandchildren informing grandparents about math test results, to speechlessness. Some people hurt so much nothing came out, except, somehow, I think I knew what they wanted to say. I could hear it in their breathing, in their tight inhalations, and though the segment didn't communicate this, I imagined people also called their own old lives, wanting to hear the way the world used to sound when it still made sense. I have the feeling old dorm room numbers were called, and childhood homes, and other numbers that have long since been disconnected but maybe, somewhere, still ring.

MAN-COMPUTER SYMBIOSIS

In 1960, J.C.R. Licklider, a psychologist and pioneer in the field of psychoacoustics, writes "Man-Computer Symbiosis." The text describes a future where humans and machines are harmoniously intertwined:

> In the anticipated symbiotic partnership, men will set the goals, formulate the hypotheses, determine the criteria, and perform the evaluations. Computing machines will do the routinizable work that must be done to prepare the way for insights and decisions in technical and scientific thinking. Preliminary analyses indicate that the symbiotic partnership will perform intellectual operations much more effectively than man alone can perform them.

ORIGIN

I was born in Los Angeles in 1982. In June of 1981, the Centers for Disease Control and Prevention observed the emergence of a new "cellular-immune dysfunction" passed via sexual contact. The findings, published in the *Morbidity and Mortality Weekly Report*, cited an unusual cluster of *Pneumocystis carinii* pneumonia (PCP) cases as the evidence for this new condition. The cluster, located in Los Angeles, was formed of five men between twenty-nine and thirty-six, all described as "active homosexuals" with no "clinically apparent underlying immunodeficiency." This was the first official account of what would become known as AIDS. During the early nineties my parents died of "AIDS-related complications."

PHOTOGRAPHS

Eight or nine years ago, at a secondhand shop on Seventh Avenue in Brooklyn, a friend and I combed through boxes of old photographs. I went elbow deep into some of them and pulled out a handful of gems. Remarkably, one of those finds has stayed with me all these years and I go back to it every now and again. "George and Dora, 1947," according to the elegant script on the back.

The two stand in front of a pale house. George has his arm around Dora's waist. Dora tilts her head toward George's shoulder. Autumn leaves spread out before them. A breeze catches the corner of Dora's skirt and lifts it in a wave above her knee, where it has remained frozen ever since.

There are few things in this world that make my heart work in that way where some small part of it, located deep within its ventricles, shifts and dislocates itself. It pumps all the time, but those subtle movements where it crawls to the front of the ribs and waits, fluttering—those moments are infrequent. Oddly, photographs trigger these rare instances. In short: a flimsy two-dimensional object can do what no living person can: incite my emotional defense mechanisms to lift. Looking at a picture I can be vulnerable and exist beyond my own chronology. I am able to achieve the age-old dream of being in two places at once.

Looking at George and Dora now, my heart does its thing. Everyone is innocent in a photograph because the future hasn't happened yet. It remains an undefined quantity hovering some-where over the horizon. Fate, chance, whatever you want to call it, is staved off for a few seconds when the shutter is depressed. George and Dora are probably gone now or dealing with the effects of age. Maybe this was their only photo together, or one of thousands. Perhaps they lost touch after that autumn afternoon, or it could be they lived together happily until George succumbed to a myocardial infarction in 1974 . . .

These possibilities churn around me like real, definite things while actual life slithers away the moment I peel open a text message. I am somehow always out of step, but a photograph offers a way out: a piece of life is sealed in an image, the image is sealed in a photograph, and I seal the photograph through my vision. I observe things in it, confirm them somehow, and while nothing ever becomes solid, I manage to at least, sometimes, catch myself.

TELEPRESENCE

Strictly speaking, nothing is happening *on* the internet. It is an arena where people recite, replicate, and broadcast information, but the events themselves happen elsewhere. Maybe you react (viscerally) to a tweet—a thought plucked out of someone's mind—but the reaction occurs in your own brain, not in a shared, breathable reality. Your reaction is to a screen and it is siphoned through a screen that removes traces of hair, skin, and teeth. Biological debris. Things indicative of a *living* presence.

Without the touchstones of biofeedback, we become apparitions. When I engage directly with someone, my physicality changes and a chemical adjustment occurs. Online nothing changes or needs to change despite the immediate connectivity, so I can't quite place or cognitively organize what is happening. This opens up a new category of experience: awash in nebulous clouds of data, I acquire a disembodied orientation, the closest frame of reference for which is that of the spirit world. Ghosts, poltergeists, wraiths, things that haunt—but we don't yet know the consequences of existing as such for extended periods of time. Top Google results for "long-term haunting" include:

Haunting Is the Newest Dating Trend You've Definitely Encountered . . .
Three Things You Can Do to Stop Being Haunted by Regret . . .
Haunted by Your Own Ghosts: Dealing with the Past and . . .

INTERGALACTIC NETWORK

In 1962, Licklider becomes the inaugural director of the Information Processing Techniques Office (IPTO) at the Advanced Research Projects Agency (ARPA) in Washington, D.C. In this new role he issues a series of visionary memos detailing an "Intergalactic Computer Network," or a global system of interconnected computers that facilitate sophisticated information exchange.

G IS FOR GUMSHOE

I have a distinct image of my mother, almost like a photograph, but then it moves. Vivian sits in bed reading, propped up by a collection of pillows. A perfect wedge of light emanating from a lamp on the nightstand catches her before spreading out over the wall. The angle of light creates a corresponding wedge of darkness above it, and for the hair of a second the two shapes are held together like a large abstract canvas. Vivian then flicks a page neatly with her index finger, and the scene ripples as if a stone had been dropped into it. After a moment, stillness resumes and my attention lands on the cover of her book, which features a large, yellow capital G. I attempt to trace the embossed curve of it with my eyes until she folds the book down on her chest and stretches her arms out to me. Then the image freezes again, in my mind's eye.

NO MATERIAL EVIDENCE EXISTS

No material evidence of viruses exists in the prehistoric record. Certain endogenous retroviral elements in the human genome are the closest approximation we have to fossils. It is not the preservation of an original virus, but of its echo cast through time; if we trace back the echo, we can (maybe) compress it back into something resembling the original sound. The human genome is 8 percent viral, which means that every time viruses have penetrated our germ line we have mutated in response to them. Our evolution has thus been driven in part by negotiating with viruses. They have changed us and we have changed them, and while nobody has any idea what any of this means, or where it will lead, our destinies spiral around each other, not unlike a double helix.

AZT

Anticancer drug azidothymidine, or AZT, is developed with a grant from the National Institutes of Health in 1964. AZT's purpose is to combat cancers caused by "environmental retroviruses," but clinical trials in mice show the drug to be ineffective. It is shelved and forgotten about for the next twenty years.

HOW TO SPEAK OF THE DEAD

To survive loss you, like the virus, must "go on," but: How to speak of the dead? What tense is appropriate to use? *We are gathered here today for our dearly*—present tense. *They were so full of life*—past tense. In the reel of my memory currently unwinding they *are* laughing—2:42 A.M. (GMT). They are ingrained in my nerves, my senses, their way of thinking siphoned through the network of my mind, their manner of speech caught swimming in my mouth— and I am still alive, still ticking, so how dead *is this really*? Aren't they still echoing through my DNA?

THE PARTY

My parents met at a party in Santa Monica or Venice. It was a new, money-filled decade. It was summer. The sun shone in the sky for twelve hours straight.

Recently divorced, she drove a midnight-colored Porsche. She was older than she looked, and was pursuing a second (or third?) degree in psychology/public health at UCLA. He had left the UK because he was in trouble with the law. He sported a mustache and was taller than almost every other man in the room.

They exchanged some words, which led to a casual relationship, which led to a weekend in Vegas, which led to me, which led to them both being dead a few years later, at the beginning of another decade.

I don't know how I know about the party, or the trouble with the law. I don't even know if any of these things are true or if I fabricated them over time—except, I do know about the Porsche, and the affiliation with UCLA, and the weather. The weather, at least, hasn't changed. The sun still burns.

A CONTINUOUS LINE

What is a lineage? A "continuous line of descent"? A downward cascade of information? A passage of traits lowered from point A to point B? We conceive of lineage as the most basic of geometric forms, but inherited characteristics alter as they pass in and out of flesh, as well as time, and: Isn't a line actually representative of un-changing circumstances? Doesn't it just show, on closer inspection, the perpetuation of a singular configuration—a point—simply shifting through space?

GEMMA

I listened to the story of the phone booth at work. I was stationed in the attic that afternoon so I let it play freely off my phone know-ing I would be alone for several hours. I had been tasked with hand rolling three hundred posters and stuffing them into tubes that would be mailed to shops across the UK for the promotion of a new product. It was a thankless, mindless job, but I was ever grate-ful for it, always keeping at the back of my mind a list of truly mis-erable professions I could be doing, and for less money.

When Gemma showed up to evaluate my progress, I had the legs of the story running through me. I saw her ebullient, curly bob bounce up from the spiral staircase and all the feelings that had surfaced during the last twenty minutes instantly dissolved. She stayed for the better part of her lunch break to "help" me because she found some aspect of my performance unsatisfactory. The only deficiency I could identify was simply the fact that I was doing it and not her.

While we rolled and stuffed I did my best to lay out a series of pleasantries I hoped might evolve into a stream of conversation. After several dead ends, we eventually fell into a rhythm where I asked a question and she would provide me with an exceptionally long and detailed answer, almost like an etching. From this I learned that Gemma was going through the migraines of home renovations: her kitchen was "in a state" due to the installation of under-floor heating, which not only displaced the rhythms of the household with her children and husband but caused nerve-shredding noise. I wanted to ask what sort of hours the contractors were keeping because I couldn't figure out when she would be around to hear any of it since she was always at the office, but I refrained. I attempted to lighten the mood by bringing up how exquisite her feet would feel come winter, but she could only respond by remixing all she had said before, finishing off with the phrase "This is the worst thing ever."

I endeavored to take her seriously. I wanted to absorb what she was saying through my skin and hold it as a delicate confidence someone had entrusted me with, but I could not. Instead, I kept thinking about the phone booth, the wind telephone, they called it, and how it would feel to lift the receiver. I kept thinking about how the line from living to dead is just that, a line, the smallest of separations.

MESSAGE BLOCKS

In 1964, engineer Paul Baran, working for the RAND Corporation, designs a communications system capable of surviving a nuclear attack. Unlike telephony, his system does not work through pointed, centralized channels, but through a dendritic network that allows information to be spontaneously rerouted via different pathways. Crucially, information is transmitted via "blocks"; this means messages are segmented into smaller units of communication in order to travel more efficiently through the network. Baran refers to this concept, rather unimaginatively, as "message blocks."

RECORD OF THOUGHT

Music and photo albums appeal to different sensory faculties but their purposes are the same: to present a record of thought. An album, regardless of species, crushes experience into matter. The raw data of a life is converted into a visual/aural document for safekeeping, but in the face of everything, what could be a more feeble gesture? Doesn't an album just show how we try to hold on to the things that leave us, and don't they just leave anyway?

MINITEL

The Minitel was an "electronic phone book" popular in France during the eighties and nineties. It consisted of a CRT monitor and keyboard that could be plugged directly into a telephone jack. In other words: it was a primitive PC with online capabilities. The device was launched by the government in response to a report titled "The Computerization of Society" (1978), which provided a grim analysis of the French technosphere. Widely recognized at the time for having the worst telephone network "in the industrialized world," the report advised digitizing phone lines and overlaying them with a graphical interface. The logic behind the inclusion of visual information was to rouse citizen engagement, drawing attention to the wonder of French innovation and reemphasizing its place within cultural identity; the report also begrudgingly acknowledged the increased presence of American tech in the workplace. The tonic for all these issues was believed to be the Minitel, which would also eliminate the extravagant cost of annual phone book reprints. While constructing a machine for mass distribution was perhaps an idiosyncratic solution to save on paper costs, it was one heavily flavored by the era's enthusiasm for telematics, "a combination of telecommunications and informatics." The future, if it was anywhere, was flowing over screens.

Minitels were free and made widely available. Usage, however, was charged per minute at fluctuating price points. Once logged in, typical phone book information appeared along with cinema times, weather reports, stock prices, and personal banking information. Certain features could even handle "natural language requests," which enabled users to to purchase theater tickets or make train reservations in real time. Despite this particular advancement, there was no "app" that facilitated peer-to-peer communication until a teen hacker took it upon himself to develop something akin to AOL Instant Messenger, or so the story goes. The renegade feature caught on like wildfire and became so popular it was formalized within the network. Official chat rooms were born. Unsurprisingly, as humans were involved in this endeavor, a great number of these chat rooms took on an illicit bent. An adult-themed subculture called Minitel Rose, or Pink Minitel, emerged, and, without question, became Minitel's most lucrative aspect. An entirely new workforce blossomed to man it. People were hired to impersonate ladies of the night and to message with customers for as long as possible. Sexual chat went by the name of "messageries roses."

As the internet and World Wide Web rose to prominence, the Minitel faded, with senior citizens becoming the device's primary demographic. However, it survived until 2012, such was its popularity.

MYSTERY!

Every parental figure or guardian has their own set of fixations locked inside objects left round the house. These objects are evidence of a private life in which you play no part. The framed concert posters, pine cone collections, matryoshka dolls, amps, gardening tools, and vintage whiskeys are germs of an autonomous, adult identity, and yet these germs leach out into the environment. As a child you absorb them. They inform your visual field.

When I try to think of Vivian as a person and not as a mother or wife, I scan our household and look at the shelves. I study the contents of her closet, leaf through her suits. I examine the cassette tapes she organized by color. I scratch at my memory for what held her attention, and I circle back again and again to the stack of paperbacks she kept on her bedside table. All mysteries written by Agatha Christie, Tony Hillerman, and Sue Grafton. These were the books she read for pleasure and so she kept them close. They did not cross the threshold of the living room to be displayed alongside *Bulfinch's Mythology* or *The Hero with a Thousand Faces,* but as far as I know, this wasn't for appearances' sake because as I continue to glide through the memories of this period, I see that when she wasn't reading mysteries they were playing on our television. Essentially, if a show had a case to solve, even if it was medical in nature (*Diagnosis: Murder*), chances are Vivian had it on as a background track while she balanced her checkbook at the dining room table. The courtroom/cop variety were fixtures of daytime programming, while the armchair detectives dominated the evenings. Reruns of *Perry Mason* filled the late afternoons, its black-and-white images ran disconnected in front of my eyes. Something about the show's lack of color made it impossible for me to latch on to faces and so the plots became impenetrable. The only discernible feature of the experience was the theme tune with its dramatic brass overture blowing a few ominous notes before dissolving into a melody that invoked the feeling of swirling a scotch at five o'clock.

I start to hum the tune now and slowly ease myself out of memory lane and into research mode. I google *Perry Mason* and read several episode recaps. From what I can gather they follow a strict formula: Week after week, in the city of Los Angeles, criminal defense attorney Mason takes on a client falsely accused of murder. An investigation is carried out, shenanigans ensue, and then in a climactic courtroom scene Mason unmasks the real killer, inevitably on the witness stand. Mason's client is thus exonerated, and everyone goes home happy. Wikipedia notes that the closing line of each episode is always a "humorous remark." I now understand why the show may have been ideal for a young viewer.

Televised mysteries are, by nature, preposterous. How events are dramatized to operatic levels and then dropped neatly into a fortuitous sequence is so unlike anything in real life it's basically comedy. Despite any wrong turns or false leads the plot nevertheless moves forward. Then there are the exposition sequences where, always in front of an audience, the detective reconstructs the crime narrative for the sake of the audience at home. For a brief moment *Murder, She Wrote* flickers in my mind. While not quite as predictable as *Mason,* certain elements appeared with such frequency that my grandmother Nivia once remarked, "I'm never inviting that woman to dinner," because people were constantly getting offed at the dinner parties Mrs. Fletcher was attending. But this is exactly what I mean: why does the murder always occur where the detective happens to be dining? And beyond these improbable conveniences, there are the detectives themselves to contend with: Poirot with his unusual clipped gait, the refined yet restrained Miss Marple, the married duo Tommy and Tuppence, in search of adventure and money . . .

I remember these eccentrics from *Mystery!* on PBS along with muted color palettes, and gray London light filtering through drawing rooms, setting them into a pearlescent murk. But more so, underneath this, are the shivering lines of Edward Gorey's intro animation for the series. I pull it up on YouTube and watch the black ink strokes carve out a sequence of mutating scenes: a pterodactyl flies out of an urn, lightning bolts erupt from a densely thatched sky, and a gravestone cracks into pieces as a widow figure casually sips a glass of red wine beside it. Next, a trio of coppers walk on tiptoe swinging their flashlight beams into the dark, only to accidentally discover a pair of legs sinking into a pond . . . I feel the memory of these pictures echo fathoms below my skin.

I quit my browser and stare at the high-res nebula on my desktop. What was Vivian's attraction to this genre? If I could know this, then perhaps I could know something of her thoughts. Was it the distraction that appealed to her, or the strange absorption these stories offered? Mysteries have the curious effect of pulling you in before you're aware of it. Suddenly you're inside the plot without having made any clear decision to get involved. The reaction is automatic. Our brains seem wired to correct the disturbance caused by a mystery right alongside the detective. Perhaps this is what the popularity of the genre ultimately reveals: a cognitive predisposition toward balance, maybe even harmony.

Metaphors also point toward this tendency. The configuration of a metaphor forces a misalignment of ideas which irritates the mind; unable to fluidly classify its components the mind is provoked, unwittingly, to resolve the glitch of information. In doing so, the meaning of "all the world's a stage," or "heart of stone," emerges, although not in words. Strictly speaking, the meaning of a metaphor doesn't exist on the page. It resides only in thought, and when we catch ourselves moving through our thoughts and discovering the meaning, it creates a small moment of effervescence, of delight.

RADIOLAB HIV

On Sundays when there is nothing to do and my phone looks like a limp creature jacked into the wall that will never ping or vibrate ever again, I listen to podcasts to pass the time. Today's selection is about a scratch, a splitting of the epidermis that occurred 120 years ago. The setting for the event was a stretch of rainforest in southeast Cameroon measuring approximately one hundred square miles. Enclosed by three rivers and a mountain range, the territory was virtually isolated from the rest of the world except via waterway. According to the podcast, it was here, over a century ago, where a hunter floated downstream, perhaps on a canoe, and made landfall. He then entered the forest and proceeded to execute the tasks of his profession, including the slaughter of a chimpanzee. It is inferred that during the hunting or butchering process, the hunter cut himself and blood from the chimp's carcass dripped or "spilled over" into this abrasion. Along with the chimp's blood, however, came a virus. As the genomes of humans and primates are nearly identical, the virus barely had to adapt to survive. Simian immunodeficiency virus simply mutated into human immunodeficiency virus. When the hunter returned to civilization, he brought this new viral strain with him, where it now had infinite vectors to spread . . .

A cut to a hunter must be an occupational hazard so common it escapes perception, and yet, to think the whole world turned on something perhaps no larger than an eyelash crushes the air right out of my lungs. I need a moment to search for my breath, but the podcast hosts steamroll on, unfazed, tracing the fateful SIV spillover strain back to *its* genesis, to find the "true origin" of the human pandemic. After an intensive search, the strain is located, plucked apart, and analyzed by scientists worldwide. But of course, there's a twist: the analysis reveals two other strains of SIV embedded within the genome of the origin strain. This finding leads to yet another theory:

At some point in the last ten thousand years, a chimpanzee ate a small monkey known as a red-capped mangabey. The mangabey was infected with a strain of SIV specific to mangabeys, and this strain crept into the chimp during consumption, thereby infecting it. Later, hungry again, the same chimp went to town on another small monkey, a spot-nosed guenon, which just so happened to be infected with a spot-nosed-guenon-specific strain of SIV. The chimp then became infected with the guenon strain, making it simultaneously host to two *different strains of the same virus. This isn't even the batshit crazy part. Apparently, things like this happen all the time. The anomaly here is that both viral strains end up inhabiting the same cell, and during the viral replication process the cell inadver-*

tently mixes up code from the mangabey strain and the guenon strain, resulting in a hybrid virus.

The thing about hybrid viruses is that "99.9999 percent of the time" they are completely worthless. Their remixed code either produces a lame-ass virus the host can instantly crush or nothing at all. The probability of a hybrid virus landing on "the exact combination of factors for it to evade the host's immune system" is exceedingly rare, or "a blue moon, in a blue moon, in a blue moon."

PACKET SWITCHING

In 1965, at the National Physical Laboratory in the UK, computer scientist Donald Davies develops "packet switching," a concept that coincidentally resembles Baran's "message blocks." In Davies's iteration, a computer message is divided into "packets" that are distributed along pathways of a network before reconfiguring at their destination. Through consultation with a linguist, Davies selects the word "packet" for his invention, as it seamlessly translates into several languages with little conceptual loss. Packet switching eventually overtakes message blocks as industry standard.

TRANSFERENCE OF ENERGY

In *Madness, Rack, and Honey,* poet Mary Ruefle focuses on the concept of metaphor. From her perspective, "Metaphor is not, and never has been, a mere literary term," but is "an event." She goes on: "*A poem must rival a physical experience* and metaphor is, simply, an exchange of energy between two things." In other words, for a poem to challenge everyday living it must unfold within time the same way as a football match or a date. A poem must *happen,* and metaphor is the instrument by which this is possible precisely because it occurs over time: there is the time it takes to observe a metaphor, and the time it takes to cognitively assemble it. The transference of energy thus happens both within the text in its lines and outside of it, in the brain. The "event" is that of the words moving across the mind's eye.

Ruefle continues:

> If you believe that metaphor is an event, and not just a literary term denoting comparison, then you must conclude that a certain philosophy arises: the philosophy that everything in the world is connected. I'll go slowly here: if metaphor is not idle comparison, but an exchange of energy, an event, then it unites the world by its very premise—that things connect and exchange energy. And if you extrapolate this philosophy further, you eventually cease to believe in separate realities.

In other words: energy cannot be created or destroyed. It just moves between things in the universe. By understanding ideas through metaphor, loose dimensions of experience are woven together. The past comes back.

YOUR MEMORY'S NATURAL ORGANIZATION

1. Sometimes the only way to say something is to say it. To condense it into prose or thicken it with style will chemically alter it, and the point really is to communicate, to share an idea.

2. When we say a disease is "communicable" it is another way of saying it is transmissible via casual contact. It can be shared

between people like a dinner bill or an Uber ride, and also a file attachment or a meme.

3. HIV is the most intimate of viruses. The exchange of it relies on sex, blood, and needles, three things most people avoid talking about unless it's life-or-death.

4. Blood is liquid that, outside of its container, sticks to surfaces. The stain of it is hard to erase, like a jagged remark caught on the edge of the ear. Both linger and contain oxygen, and sometimes they both contain lead.

5. Nosebleeds are common at high altitudes, as are shortness of breath, dizziness, and nausea. The pressure of the body changes at around eight thousand feet, which at one point was sea level.

6. People climb mountains to crush their limitations. They do it for novelty and adrenaline, but they also do it to be put in their place: sure, you can scale a peak, stand triumphantly on a summit, and smile, but doesn't that just show you how small you are compared to everything else?

7. It took humans a while to convey perspective in visual art. For thousands of years, everything was flat and existed on a single plane. There was no way to represent distance between objects other than to reduce or enlarge their size, which, without a vanishing point, created unintentionally eerie scenes.

8. There is a scene in a TV show where a duck swims around in a condo bathtub. The thirty-two-year-old son, with dark curls

and a moody disposition, has come to visit his mother. The mother is out brunching "with the girls," and the large, burly, ponytailed boyfriend of the mother answers the door. It is awkward between them but, before it gets too difficult, the two hear distressed quacking outside. Cut to: the duck in the bathtub with the two men staring at it. The son says, "I thought stuff would be adding up by now, but it's like everything's slipping through," to which the boyfriend says, "Can I say something?" and the conversation turns to grief. The son's biological father has recently transitioned into womanhood. The father isn't dead, but is no longer The Father, which is hard for the son to grasp. The son remarks that it is not "politically correct to say you've missed someone who has transitioned."

BOYFRIEND: This isn't about correct. This is about grieving. Mourning. Have you mourned the loss of your father?
SON: I did not like him.
BOYFRIEND: So?
SON: I don't know how to do that.

The son then breaks down sobbing as the boyfriend enshrines him in a bear hug. Meanwhile, in the background, the duck quietly glides by.

9. Experience is difficult to discuss because it rests in tissue, in neural pathways. It is a biochemical situation that moves like liquid in a skin suit. There's no language there. No means of transmission or spread, only bones, veins, and muscle.

10. Another way of considering scale: the skeleton of a brontosaurus suspended in a cavernous atrium with a child below it, pointing.

11. In Rainer Maria Rilke's only novel there is a passage that reads:

Is it possible . . . that no one has seen or recognized or said anything that's real and important? Is it possible that there have been thousands of years in which to look, to reflect, and to record, and that these thousands of years have been allowed to go by like a school break when one eats a sandwich and an apple?

12. Yeah, dude. It's totally possible.

13. *Guinness World Records* lists the Makhonjwa Mountains as the oldest mountain range in the world. Its age: 3.6 billion years old; its highest peak: 5,905 feet.

14. Time can be measured in what you do not do with it and what you do not say in it. Time can be measured, in other words, by nothing at all.

15.

BLUE MOON

It is difficult to pinpoint the exact occurrence rate of a blue moon because the concept has a checkered past. According to *The Maine Farmers' Almanac*, which began publication in 1819, a blue moon was considered the third full moon in a season of four. This concept stood for 118 years, until a famed misinterpretation of the 1937 edition of the *Almanac* was written up by James Hugh Pruett. Through some unfortunate calculation Pruett took the *Almanac*'s view to mean that a blue moon was the second full moon in a month. How he arrived at this conclusion is anyone's guess, but it oddly became the go-to blue moon definition that was then published for many years. It was then further popularized in an influential volume of *Sky & Telescope* magazine in 1946, which was cited throughout the decades, most notably on an episode of the radio show *StarDate* in 1980. These inconsistencies have persisted, alongside the idiom of improbability, "once in a blue moon." And then of course, there is the observed atmospheric phenomenon wherein smoke and dust particles of a very particular size rise up from the Earth and cast the moon in blue overtones. All this being said, determining the probability of "a blue moon, in a blue moon, in a blue moon" defies all calculation.

LO FOR LOGIN

The Advanced Research Projects Agency Network, or ARPANET, commissioned by the US Department of Defense, is launched in 1969. It is a realization of Licklider's Intergalactic Computer Network and links four academic institutions—University of California, Los Angeles; Stanford; University of California, Santa Barbara; and the University of Utah—via Donald Davies's packet switching method. On October 29, UCLA student programmer Charley Kline contacts the Stanford Research Institute in a first attempt at messaging in real time. Unfortunately, the system crashes after Kline types in the first two characters of his text: "lo" for "login."

I WAS WRITING A BOOK

I was writing a book when my grandmother died. I was writing it because I was trying to work something out of my system, something at the very depths of it that I couldn't see but was acutely aware of resting underneath the tissues of my body. It registered only as a dull, chronic ache that increased in pressure over time to the point where living became excruciating. It took my face and pressed it into the glittering concrete, held it there until my whole life screeched to a halt, a thin trail of smoke drifting into the air behind it. I had the taste of salt in my mouth. My temperature dropped. The chemical processes within me consistently malfunctioned. I knew it was bad because I couldn't envision any sort of future for myself. I was drifting in and out of days, searching for what to do, but all the typical ways of changing one's life—extreme fitness, extreme dieting, gluttony, drugs, volunteering, imbibing, religion, hiking, marathon running, therapy, pet therapy, retail therapy, sexual addiction, overachievement, total failure—well, none of these held any appeal for me. It was only through writing that I could attempt to elucidate the matters below my vision and then try to do as everyone says: let them go. The aforementioned pursuits were simply distractions that put pain on hold, but the action of writing seemed to restore sight, or at least could make apparent what I was no longer seeing—or didn't want to see.

After a while it became clear there was no future for me because I didn't want one. An established life, with people and things in it, could be ripped away from you and seared open in such a heinous way you would never recover. You would be alive, yes, but your own breath would become a curse to you, your lungs perversely maintaining their duty for no reason at all.

But by the time I had figured this all out, my grandmother died and none of it mattered.

Nivia was ninety-three, so on some level her death had been expected for a while. In fact, I had thought about it frequently since she became my legal guardian because I knew that if I didn't hold it fixed in my mind, the thing of it, when it happened, would shatter me. I had lived with her since I was ten, and even though our relationship was a strange combination of volatile and empty, it had not been nothing. My father died in 1990, and my mother in 1993, and of the people left in my life, a smattering of aunts and uncles, Nivia was the only true adult.

It was a cerebral hemorrhage that did it. The bleeding and pressure were so severe they pushed the hemispheres of her brain off-center, toward one side of her skull.

"You should see the scan," the ICU nurse said to me. "I've never seen anything like it."

In a hospital all the layers of social veneer we struggle to uphold are unceremoniously dropped. You can just be two people in a room talking to each other. The nurse learned I was a photographer within a few minutes of my arrival so it was somehow natural to discuss images, whatever they may be, but before I could respond he had left the curtained cubicle and I never did get to see the scan.

When he returned a few hours later, he resumed our conversation as if he'd only stepped out for a second.

"So where are you from?"

"El Segundo," I said.

"Oh, you're a South Bay girl? All the other nurses said you just flew in from somewhere?"

"Yes. London."

"Oh wow. That's far."

It is far. According to Google Maps the distance between my flat in London and the Harbor-UCLA Medical Center, a hospital primarily known for treating victims of gang violence and having absurdly limited parking, is 5,452 miles. Twenty hours before this moment, I received a flurry of WhatsApp messages and eventually a phone call from Nivia's caregiver. She put me on speakerphone when the paramedics arrived, and all of the sounds were bad. Minutes later, when I shut the front door to my flat to head to the airport, I understood that on my return, there would be a different person unlocking it. I understood it in some remote way, like how you know things from watching too many movies. The accumulation of artificial experience can, after a certain point, feel like the shell of something real. Over time, the shell grows into a reference point that can be used to navigate the future despite the fact that it's fictional. When I boarded the plane, I had a montage running through my head of characters trying to resume their old lives after experiencing tragedy. None of them ever succeed. They wipe out the thing they were at the start of the film—architect, corporate lawyer, failed actor—and wind up living in a remote fishing village minding a lighthouse or starting a community garden for disadvantaged teens. They wind up taking guitar lessons like they've always dreamt about, and then play, triumphantly, at a community center open-mic night. The characters find a happiness they could never have envisaged pre-tragedy, a happiness that eclipses all they had before. They become heroes. End of story.

In my case, I had no idea what would happen because my life had no form. I took it with me place to place but I couldn't seem to make anything grow from it. My friends encouraged patience, but I blinked and ten years went by with nothing solid to show for it.

"You? Are you local?" I asked the nurse.

"Long Beach, born and raised. But I live in Torrance now."

We spoke of the beach cities of Los Angeles. Not the Malibus or Venice Beaches everyone is familiar with, but a rim of smaller places that dip south in a curve toward San Pedro. Nothing happens in any of them. Some are obscenely wealthy, some have teenagers with drug problems, others have jazz clubs. All of them contain beautiful, easy living, which is to say the problems of the greater world evaporate in their atmospheres. If there's trouble, it's ADHD or traffic. The nurse, a stocky Filipino guy with a tattoo of the Virgin Mary on his forearm, told me of his SoCal existence with a terrier mix, Dorito. While he talked, I took hold of Nivia's swollen hand and thought absolutely nothing. When I say nothing I mean every thought I had became transparent and dispersed into some weather of the mind. I could only seem to take note of her manicure: an iridescent magenta shade that reminded me of the early nineties.

The nurse turned the conversation on me. He asked a few gentle questions about El Segundo and London, and how a girl goes from life in a shitty, blue-collar, Chevron-owned town like El Segundo to London, and before I knew it, before I even had any idea words were coming out of my mouth, I unraveled my life to him as if I hadn't spoken to a soul in years. And of course, as I tell him things, I realize that I'm really telling her. He knows this, and I know this, and we both know that we both know, and she's just . . . dying, and after what feels like hours of talking, I abruptly stop because tears have started to fall out of my face as if they came from somewhere else and my face was an obstacle they had to pass through to get to their destination. I was just a thing in their way. The nurse kept adjusting tubes, taking vitals, and maneuvering around the tiny space with a grace seen only in television chefs. A box of tissues appeared at my left elbow out of thin air.

"Have you ever been to Europe? Or London?" I managed to get out, eventually.

"Well, we got perfect weather and I surf when I'm not here. My parents are still in LB and my little sister just started at UCLA . . . So I guess I just never saw the need, you know? 'Why see the world when you got the beach?' You know that Frank Ocean song?"

I nodded. I knew it.

WHAT A PICTURE CAN DO

It is sometimes very difficult to know what you are feeling. You can detect movements, perceive shifts in tension, and perhaps the volume of a feeling, but not be able to give it a name. When I look inside my own mind, I am often confronted by a wall of congealed images so thick and gray, there's no hope of getting past it, so I lift up the lid of my skull and peer downward. Inside is a goldfish bowl full of shadows that slip and slither over one another. Somehow, I understand these shadows are feelings, but just as I figure this out, they disperse into my body and form an additional membrane under my skin. In short, you can be aware that you are feeling something and not have any idea what, specifically, it is: a recipe for madness.

Enter a photograph—

Without fuss, without effort, a photograph can contain within it information that mirrors an exact feeling. The brain sees the content of the photograph and suddenly the vagueness floating inside of it acquires a form, a scene. The picture is now the feeling and photography becomes a shorthand for it. This is why it is hard to say more than "I love this" or "that's cool" when looking at a photo. Any deeper reaction plunges us back into the murk of the nervous system, where there are only temperatures and heartbeats.

TINDER MONKEY

Mark, twenty-six, is shirtless in the photo with a blue-and-white-striped towel swung over one shoulder and a monkey perched on the other. The monkey has the shriveled face of an old man, and its toothy mouth is cracked open like it's laughing, like Mark has told it the funniest joke ever, but its deft little humanlike hand is reaching out for Mark's ear like it wants to grab the ear or tear it off. Mark has no idea. He just stares into the camera grinning like a fool, the tropical sun bouncing off his perfectly capped teeth.

Every time I see one of these on Tinder my stomach churns. The idea of letting something as vile as a monkey get that close to your face is . . . unsavory. After all, monkeys and humans share 96 percent of the same genetic code and seeing that similarity in action is just plain uncanny. Animal behaviorists study groups of chimpanzees for insights into our own power structures and while these animals do participate in complex communities with rituals and hierarchies, they also possess a rabid barbarism. I once heard a story where a chimp ate an organ out of another smaller monkey, without killing the poor thing first—presumably because the tidbit tasted better fresh. Either that, or the bloodlust was the attraction, and well: Is that the 96 percent in action or the 4 percent? Who knows? So Mark advertising his skill with a wild primate really strikes me as the wrong message to send to potential mates.

But *there are so many of them.* How are there so many of them?

In general, the uniformity of men's profiles is comedy. It's as if the profile of the first man to ever get laid through the app was interpreted as a magical template and broadcast to all men everywhere. I don't doubt the women's profiles adhere to their own set of conventions, but I can guarantee there is more latitude within their interpretations than within the gentlemen's. There are days when I swipe through my feed and I feel as though I'm seeing the same guy over and over again with hardly any variation except for name. The situation echoes *Groundhog Day* except it is my life and I'm not sure how much longer my life can handle Kevin, Chad, or Steve enjoying a beach sunset in Cabo, wearing a knit beanie at Machu Picchu, or taking selfies in a public bathroom. I'm not sure how much longer my life can handle the awkward shots of Mom, or of the "mystery blonde" (is she the ex, the co-worker, the sister, the cousin?), or of the Audi/Maserati lean. My personal favorite is a phenomenon I refer to as "gay wedding," which depicts Guy in a tux with his arm around another guy in a tux after they've had a few, looking so smug and satisfied with each other's company they couldn't possibly need anyone else in the world—let alone a woman. The subsequent profile photos cast further confusion as they all contain Guy and guy with a variety of other male companions, so beyond the question of sexuality I'm never even entirely sure if I can identify which one is actually Chris, Taylor, or Justin.

The tailoring of a self for a three-second glance is utterly fascinating. I know these pictures are meant to convey sex appeal, power, wealth, athleticism, and humor, but there's no trace of a person there. All I see is a zombie consciousness, replicating a singular idea of masculinity, or what a male brain thinks women want . . . It's natural though, I guess: if you copy an image or idea of power, it feels like it's yours. You feel like you own it, if only in two dimensions. But I suppose it's even more primal than that: after all, we are animals genetically wired to conform for survival. Imitation of gestures and behaviors is encouraged, because those that can't or won't conform fall to the periphery, become outsiders, and die. Very few species survive in the wild as lone units without the support of a clan or a pride or a pack or a host, so monkey see, monkey do. Monkey—

ELECTRONIC MAIL

The first application for ARPANET is developed in 1971. It is called electronic mail, and unlike previous messaging programs, it allows users the freedom to access their communications from different terminals. To ensure messages arrive at their intended destinations, they are "addressed" with the login name of the user and the computer hostname. These are separated with the @ symbol, an innovation by computer programmer Ray Tomlinson.

THE 110 FREEWAY

The 110 freeway creates a gash in the flesh of downtown Los Angeles. The north- and southbound lanes cut through the district and sink below street level, causing chrome and glass office buildings to erupt along their sides. As a teenager, encased in the bullet of my car, racing beneath these structures at night, I was equal parts invincible and vulnerable, never quite sure where I was going, but *going*. In those few miles I embodied velocity, and after a minute or so the whole of the city would appear in my rearview as a glittering fiction, one so painfully beautiful and alluring I believed I could find love in it. A deep love. A soul love. The shimmer of those lights paused the grief that thrummed along my skull. They made me put it on the road. The mess of it hardened and I drove over it, smoothing it down into a long, thin line that stretched forever behind me.

AGE OF VIRUSES

What is the oldest terrestrial thing you can imagine? Broken cups encased in ash in Pompeii, papyrus, the gold leafing of Aztec jewelry, hieroglyphics, the mastodon? What about daisies, or red blood cells? Plankton? Freshwater amoebas? Glaciers? I guarantee we would contemplate all of these things or things like them before rabies or measles. It never occurs to us that viruses possess age. Our interest in them begins in symptoms and ends in treatment, with hardly any deviation. In fact, you probably have more immediate information about the age of your Brita filter or toothbrush than the common cold, which has been infecting people on a seasonal basis since the glory days of Cleopatra. You probably know more about some bullshit TikTok dance or the latest crypto crash than how viruses have sculpted our DNA. On the list of ancient artifacts that we might generate if asked, we would leave viruses out of it even though they have shaped our species one way or another, ever since we were a species. As Eula Biss writes in *On Immunity,*

> The cells that form the outer layer of the placenta for a human fetus bind to each other using a gene that originated, long ago, from a virus. Though many viruses cannot reproduce without us, we ourselves could not reproduce without what we have taken from them.

WRITING ABOUT DEAD PARENTS

It is hard to write about your dead parents in any way that is appropriate and yet: you must write about them. There seems to be no suitable language . . . Talking about the past turns the words im-

mediately to dust as if the tense were an incantation, a bloody en-
chantment from a fairy story. It seems easier to describe the
hammering outside or the sound of the 747 passing overhead. Writing a few lines about these brief occurrences seems easier than describing people you will never encounter because, a plane has a
future. It will land at Heathrow and people will disembark into lives
and holidays and connecting flights. Baggage will be collected, a
tear will be shed, and a dog will run around a curb while its owner
taps out a WhatsApp message. The hammering next door will turn
into a sunroom extension. By next spring, the kids will play in it,
drag in their Lego collections and spread the pieces wildly all over
the new hardwood floor.

ONE-LINER

A line can be a story you tell yourself.

INTERNETWORKING

In a technical paper written for the ARPA publication Request for
Comments (RFC) in 1974, the term "internet" emerges for the first
time. It is used as an abbreviation for "internetwork." One of its
authors, Vint Cerf, will later be recognized as one of "the fathers of
the internet."

GOING TO THE MOVIES

Nivia and I never had much in common. Our natures were carved
from different elements that, when confined to the same environment for too long, became explosive. We belonged to different

places and times and there was no way to reconcile that. Not even through love. The sixty years between us sat like a block of lead that absorbed all light and oxygen around it, decaying the atmosphere. During her lifetime the world had undergone tectonic shifts— WWII, Vietnam, the Civil Rights Movement, MLK Jr., Nixon, JFK, and the Cold War, to name a few—but the events that happened in her senior years were of something else entirely. They were different in their speed, and the velocity altered how people thought about them, wrote of them, and then before anyone could adjust to these new metrics, the transmission of information changed too. The World Wide Web ignited a big bang, a simultaneous contraction and expansion of all recorded knowledge up to that point. Scanned images of ancient manuscripts were available right alongside GeoCities pages devoted to *Dr. Quinn, Medicine Woman* fan fiction. As a teenager, having unrestricted access to this, to what felt like everything that ever was, stopped my heart. The sheer amount of information was crushing and the time of it and in it, online, was separate from real, actual geological time, which is what Nivia woke up in, worked in, and slept in.

During the AOL years she would periodically ask me to explain how email worked.

"Everyone has their own mailbox, I understand, yes. But, does it look like an actual mailbox? How is it like?"

"Yes . . . sort of. Well, there's a picture of a mailbox on the screen but—"

"Then there is the mailman? This is the computer though . . . but how does one computer deliver to another computer?"

At this point I would attempt some bullshit explanation about how computers "talked" to each other through modems, but since I barely understood it myself the conversation would rapidly deflate. Cellphones were much more concrete in her mind, though she refused to acknowledge their utility. Another phone line, whether it was connected to the land or pulsing through the air, was, at the end of the day, simply another bill.

Beyond the occasional touchstones of technology, weather, and local happenings, we spoke very little. In the aftermath of Vivian's death, there didn't seem to be anything to say. Our house would have been eerily quiet were it not for Nivia's compulsive television watching, the sounds of fake families filling in our own empty rooms. In the kitchen there was an old black-and-white set with a twist dial that refused to die, so Nivia kept it on the counter where it was nearly always within her arm's reach. The living room was organized around a large black Zenith that felt rather space-age against her floral décor, its lightning-bolt logo a searing call from the future. A new twenty-inch bought on installments from Best Buy lived in her bedroom, and one that essentially functioned as a radio was stationed in the garage, its picture surfacing only occasionally from an ocean of monochrome static. Frequently, two or more of these sets were on simultaneously, tuned to the same station, a slight echo occurring between them. This shifted at nighttime when she watched her prime-time dramas alone in the living room with the lights off. From the street she appeared to be in a fish tank, the strange electronic hues moving in waves around her motionless body. Lately, now, whenever I find myself passing by a flat late at night and see a TV casting broad shadows along the wall of a room, my heart hurts.

The only thing left for two people to talk about in a situation like this is culture, at least some small sliver of it, and our one point of contact became the cinema, inevitable perhaps for two lost souls in Los Angeles. We had nothing and so our geographic circumstances filtered through us until we too dreamed of the screen, like all the other fools who came before us.

Sitting in the dark for two-hour intervals chipped away enough of the day that some of the pressure between us was relieved. We left the shells of our lives out in the parking lot and surrendered to the ones happening onscreen. A film would fold us into its plotline and while we both had wildly separate experiences of those scripted events, at least we were next to each other as they happened. When the last credits rolled off the screen and the lights came on we would drift slowly back to the car and talk. We finally had something to talk about.

For some reason, when I think back to this time, it is always summer and school is out. I see us ride up the glass elevator to the top floor of the South Bay Galleria and stroll underneath fake palm fronds and skylights to the entrance of the GC Multiplex. Outside the sun is a million degrees but inside the air-conditioning stings, puckering our skin. The scent of burnt buttered popcorn emanates from the concession stand across the lobby, and teenagers wearing uniforms of mustard and purple awkwardly manage the ticket lines. Around us, people are excited about "the big screen" and "blockbusters." People still believe in the stories they tell, and eagerly anticipate them. What I mean is, life is not yet so confusing as to render moviegoing an antiquated experience.

Nivia and I went to the movies religiously and observed rituals surrounding our visits. We would pick up a made-to-order deli sandwich from a Ralphs or Albertsons, sneak it into the theater, and share it over the trailers. The sandwich was always the same (turkey, Alpine Lace Swiss, lettuce, tomato, mayo, mustard, French roll), as was where we sat (center back). Double features were coordinated during awards season and on brutally hot afternoons. Time would evaporate completely, and before we knew it we were back in our Nissan Sentra driving home talking about Robert De Niro's physical acting in *Flawless*, how weak *You've Got Mail* was compared to *Sleepless in Seattle*, or Drew Barrymore's wondrous plaits in *Ever After*. This last film in particular stands out in my memory, though not on account of its craft or technical elements. I remember it for reasons rather difficult to explain. Nivia enjoyed it because she was pleased to see "Drew" looking so "healthy after years of messing around with drugs and boys." Her comment meant nothing to me as I didn't follow celebrity gossip and had never bothered with *E.T.*, but I could recognize that Barrymore did authentically radiate in the picture. It was something completely unrelated to her performance and had little to do with the craft of acting. The camera seemed to activate a marker in her genetic code that caused her to shimmer like she *was* Cinema, as if cinema were a quality or a condition of being. Mostly we consider cinematic and photographic spaces as areas of fabrication, but maybe this is just an easy reading of these situations. Maybe certain people can only make sense in front of a camera. Perhaps pictures, moving or otherwise, are the only places where some people can actually live, and maybe that's why, years later, I had to study photography.

PAINTINGS IN A HOSPITAL

I look back and try to remember the artwork that decorated the ICU waiting room and corridors, but the images disintegrate as if buckets of water had been splashed on them. The colors thin out, desaturate, and slide out of frame, pulling with them the forms and figures they once composed. All I seem to have retained is an overwhelming sense of familiarity, which leads me to believe they were the usual suspects: Monet's *Water Lilies,* Van Gogh's *Sunflowers,* Picasso's *Mains aux Fleurs,* but I cannot say exactly. I can tell you their locations within the ward, and describe the type of bolt used to keep their frames on the wall. I can tell you about traces of dust and patches of sun damage. I can even remember the dried body of a moth caught behind an acrylic pane, but as to the content? There seems to be a slow-motion heist going on in my memory.

There is so little to look at in a hospital, in a patient's room, that any image gives you a place to go infinitely more interesting and beautiful than the current surroundings. They become fixtures for contemplation, screens effectively inviting remembrances, hallucinations, daydreams, and associations. They serve as gateways out of time, but the main thing is they keep you company. Art in the real world, set free from the captivity of a gallery or museum and placed in the wild of an office or hotel lobby, shows you its strength. As it becomes part of your landscape it doesn't so much blend into the setting as it becomes something that helps living. It holds you in place. You're in a relationship with it regardless of how much or little you notice it because it is there unequivocally. It sees your sorrows.

LITTLE RED RIDING HOOD

The Wikipedia entry for "viral phenomenon" features a nineteenth-century illustration of Little Red Riding Hood standing under a perfect archway of trees. Behind her is a blue, open sky symbolizing freedom. Below her is the wolf, wrapped around her legs. Draped in her iconic gear, she peers down at him and he looks up at her, their interlocked gaze emphasizing their ill-fated magnetism. The wolf's jaws are ever so slightly ajar, as if he's whispering a charming greeting or a hypnotic spell. The caption reads, "Red Riding Hood, an example of a folktale."

This delicate image introduces the "History of Content Sharing" section, and in the subheading marked "Early History," the text explains, "Before writing . . . the dominant means of spreading memes was oral culture like folk tales, folk songs, and oral poetry, which mutated over time as each retelling presented an opportunity for change."

The use of the word "meme" here is harrowing. To retroactively imbue history with terms like "meme" and "selfie" puts me in a sort of terror; by doing so we lose distinctive conceptions of narrative and transmission, which is to say: we lose how people thought of life in their own time. Something deeply irrevocable, but all this aside: *Why this image?* Why Red Riding Hood? The arrangement of the headings and image on the page makes me read the situation as a metaphor and after all, isn't the tale about an innocent getting devoured? Little Red, beguiled by the wolf, surrenders all her personal information to him, and then he uses it all against her to *consume her*. The creature uses it to *literally eat her,* and all I can think is: Is this us? Is viral culture one day going to use everything we have ever put into it and eat our faces off? And then I remember: the wolf ate Grandma too.

SLIM DISEASE

Surges of a mysterious "wasting sickness" or "slim disease" are reported by hospitals throughout sub-Saharan Africa in the mid-1970s.

A PLOT OF ATMOSPHERIC IMPRESSIONS

The stories of noir fiction are bleak in vibe with plots that never quite materialize. The reader is so embedded within the detective's subjective experience of a case that a plot will only ever appear as a series of atmospheric impressions, which is a lot like how a city first appears when you drive through it at night, at age sixteen, not knowing what to do with yourself. The style and the glamour and the horror and the promise all streak through your peripheral vision, but none of it solidifies, becomes anything of import. It just remains a landscape to pass through, to pass the time away.

TOBACCO MOSAIC VIRUS

According to Google, the "first virus to be discovered" was tobacco mosaic virus (TMV). The name derives from the telltale mark of infection: an alternating pattern of light and dark splotches found exclusively on leaves. Initially known as "mosaic disease," the virus had been in circulation for hundreds of years but grew particularly rampant during the nineteenth century with frequent outbreaks occuring across Northern Europe and Russia. As tobacco was a major linchpin of these economies, eradicating the disease permanently became a matter of governmental interest. At the time, general consensus held the disease was caused by a toxin.

The connection between germs and illness was still a relatively new concept. Previously, illness had been constituted in terms of morality, dictated by the "pureness" of one's soul. The cognitive leap required to surpass this belief and get to science was colossal but German biologist Robert Koch managed it spectacularly in 1890. Koch created a series of postulates that employed logic to establish a causative relationship between pathogen and symptom. They read:

1. The microorganism must be found in abundance in all organisms suffering from the disease, but should not be found in healthy organisms.
2. The microorganism must be isolated from a diseased organism and grown in pure culture.
3. The cultured microorganism should cause disease when introduced into a healthy organism.
4. The microorganism must be re-isolated from the inoculated, diseased experimental host and identified as being identical to the original specific causative agent.

While the postulates appear comprehensive, they only apply to the range of the germ spectrum visible to nineteenth-century lab equipment. Viruses unfortunately did not fall into this category. They could not yet be imaged with microscopes, nor could they be grown artificially in a lab. Consequently, Koch's postulates were tailored toward bacterial pathogens, and had a wonderful success rate at identifying infectious agents such as anthrax. Mosaic disease, on the other hand, remained elusive, hence the rationale of labeling it something vague, like a toxin.

Though a body of evidence grew to support the existence of a new type of pathogen, there was great reluctance within the scientific community to acknowledge it. The postulates had proved triumphant over some important medical mysteries, and to go against the grain of what had quickly been adopted as industry standard carried significant professional risk. Therefore, any time a diagnostic anomaly was encountered it was quite simply shoehorned into a bacterial context. In essence, Koch's postulates shaped thought in such a way that they altered perception, narrowing the field of infectious agents down to just one.

In 1879, German agriculturist and chemist Adolf Mayer began his study of mosaic disease. While he conducted comprehensive chemical breakdowns of soil compositions and tobacco plants, the disease agent evaded him. His one discovery revolved around sap: he observed that sap taken from infected plants would transmit the disease when applied to healthy plants. As he had no way to explain this, Koch's postulates being of no help, he simply reaffirmed the source of the disease as a toxin. In time, Mayer explained, powerful "optical microscopy" would confirm the existence of this toxin, though he knew such a development was at least several decades away.

In the late 1890s, botanist Dmitri Ivanovsky was commissioned by the Russian government to locate the source of three geographically disparate mosaic disease outbreaks. Inspired by the work of Mayer, Ivanovsky conducted a series of his own sap experiments focusing on filtration. He ground infected leaves into a serum and filtered the sap-like liquid through delicate, unglazed porcelain. Filtration was upheld as the ultimate procedure for removing toxins from liquid substances, and porcelain filters, a.k.a. Chamberland filters, had proven so effective at their job it never occurred to anyone that unknown, smaller toxins could potentially exist. Ivanovsky had assumed the filtered serum would be disease-free, but when he applied it to leaves of healthy plants, they became infected. This was confounding. The findings clearly pointed toward the existence of a non-bacterial pathogen as the source of the disease, but Ivanovsky was still very much under the chokehold of the Koch postulates. That his research ran "contrary to all accepted scientific belief" did not sit well with him, so he twisted his findings into a narrative consistent with the accepted view of his era. He proposed the disease-causing entity was a "filterable agent," most likely a "toxic by-product" of submicroscopic bacterial substance, that with time would be discovered.

Everything changed in 1898 when Dutch microbiologist Martinus Beijerinck began working with TMV. As a former colleague of Mayer, he felt something of an obligation to carry on his legacy, and in doing so, came away with a unique insight: Beijerinck witnessed the disease spread through new plant growth. If mosaic disease was truly caused by a toxin or toxic by-product, its potency would diminish over time, growing weaker as the plant grew larger. He reasoned that the pathogenic element had to be something that could multiply within the plant and move through it, like a liquid. He conceptualized the germ as a "contagium vivum fluidum," or contagious living fluid. Beijerinck's insight allowed him to break out of the status quo and establish what would become modern virology. Interestingly, he believed the contagious fluid was "living" because it spread—

GO WEST

In the summer of 1967 Vivian drove to California in a pink convertible. She left New York with Dennis, her boyfriend, and Karen, her close college friend. The trio were running away from a future in a city where the cycles of heat and ice threatened a calcification of the soul they were not yet prepared to accept, so they chased the sunset to its end. They drove through the arteries of the country and into new lives they hoped would be tinged with fresh air and apricot skies.

Vivian, Dennis, and Karen arrived at a house in Hermosa Beach, situated coincidentally on Manhattan Avenue. They crashed there temporarily, but Karen soon left for the redwood trees upstate, already weary of LA's skin-deep glare. Vivian and Dennis remained in LA but left each other. Dennis had been a cop in New York City and reasoned he could be a cop in any city as long as that city had Vivian in it. Everyone thought they were destined for marriage. Everyone was wrong.

Sometimes when I catch a police drama on TV playing in a bar or in a hotel room, Dennis comes into my mind. The thoughts around him are still and simple: I just want to know if he found love again, or at least if he loved LA.

These stories have to have a happy ending at some point.

WHERE THE TWO FORCES MEET

1. The convergence of the material and immaterial occurs in the space of the album. The two forces meet there, the preserved items serving as fossils of histories, thought processes, and cardiovascular systems that have grown so porous as to be nonexistent.

2. We are physically dense entities and perhaps because of this, we show preference for things of density. The immaterial troubles us, we don't quite know what to do with it. Even kids, who are architects with thin air, forging castles and friends from it, crave the real thing, crave what they can see.

YOURS TRULY

Queen Elizabeth II becomes the first head of state to send an email in 1976. The email heralds the launch of a "new programming language," and it is signed "Elizabeth R," which remains her electronic signature for the entirety of her life.

HOW YOU GET TO BE THE WAY YOU ARE

A song enters your heart like an arrow and your psyche envelops its vector, folding it down and compressing it until it is part of your code.

IT RUNS IN THE FAMILY

Nivia once told me about visiting a medium in Canyon Country. The story was triggered by a series of sneezes that issued from my rearrangement of her closet. I was pulling ancient dry cleaning (still encased in plastic sheaths) from the back and circulating it to the front when I managed to inhale a curtain of dust. A sequence of tiny fireworks exploded from my nostrils and Nivia rushed to produce a tissue, searching a variety of compartments in her clothing and purse in effort to locate one. After the chaos subsided, she sat on the edge of the bed and swung her feet above the carpet in the manner of a little girl. I turned back in to the closet and just as I was growing accustomed to the silence, she launched into the tale of the psychic who, within moments of "contacting The Other Side," began a sneezing fit that lasted over a minute. "You've got an Indian with you," he said. "Indians make my nose itch." He was, apparently, referring to one of her "spirit guides," of which there were three—but before I could clarify if he meant a Native American or actual Indian, or ask about the term "spirit guide," or what Nivia was doing getting her fortune told in the first place, the conversation changed to another tangential reminiscence about our bloodline.

"We have a gift," she said.

"What do you mean?"

"It runs in the family."

"Like a disease?"

"No, we see things . . . We know a thing before it happens sometimes . . ."

Sure. Entirely absorbed by blazers and silk blouses I allowed myself a deeply luxurious eye roll, not that she would have seen it had we been face-to-face. A few years ago she had been declared legally blind. She suffered from macular degeneration in her left eye and the corrective surgery for the ailment shredded her remaining vision with scar tissue. She could see, but only as if through a net, and details like faces were lost entirely.

"My brother Whistle had it—"

While I continued to sort out long-sleeved blouses from short-sleeved blouses, winter skirts from summer skirts, she described branches of our family tree, providing vague histories of distant relations in Puerto Rican villages who had what some refer to as the second sight.

"Fonesito saw scenes on his television, like on a program, but the television was not running. He watched people we knew . . ."

I did my best to listen, but in those days at least half of my mind was somewhere else, usually Europe, imagining cobblestone streets and endless cafés on Parisian canals. I was dreaming of fresh baguettes strapped to bicycles, marinière shirts, and rows of wine bottles neatly arranged in shop windows, catching the late afternoon light. I longed for cities that contained shards of beauty intentionally placed to interrupt the flow of reality. This was my second sight: envisioning different circumstances under which I might flourish because the ones I was in felt like a gloved hand over my throat.

Nivia was, and continues to be, the hardest human I have ever known. She had a surgical way of extracting the ugliness from any hopeful situation in one's life and highlighting it in such a way that your love or wonder of the activity would wither away and die. It was a strange magic. Suddenly, you could not unsee what she saw even though you knew there might not be a single element of truth to it. This influence was terrifying because there was no logical reason for its potency. Oftentimes she would describe a bleak picture of my own future as if divining it straight from the air in front of her: in her estimation I was always but one step away from dancing at a topless bar on Century Boulevard. It was completely absurd, but I found myself living in perpetual fear of such a fate.

It perhaps goes without saying that Nivia had no time for poetry, and in fact, in my whole time of knowing her she never once touched a work of fiction. She viewed it as a waste of time, and based on this alone you can see that there was never any hope for us.

ELF PHOTO

Buried within Nivia's archives is a matte eight-by-ten photo of a high school drama production. It depicts a scene from a holiday review. The façades of storefronts and porches are strewn with snow, and cardboard candy canes decorate various nooks of the stage with a certain jolliness reserved only for the midfifties. On the left-hand side of the frame is Vivian dressed as an elf. Her shoes curl back on themselves with bells on the end, her hat is pointed. She escorts a girl in a hoopskirt by the hand and waist, like a gentleman, and in fact, all the other elves in the photo are men. A semicircle of elf-and-hoopskirt couples fills the apron of the stage in the approximation of a waltz or cotillion. I can only surmise that Vivian was cast in this particular role on account of her height and lack of male participation in the production, but it doesn't really matter because she completely and unequivocally glows. Her chest is lifted, her shoulder blades cascade down her back, she eclipses everything around her, but it's not to do with "stage presence" or physical beauty. It is something far stranger and more unsettling than the cut of a cheekbone, or the shape of a nose. It is the look of someone who loves living with her whole life stretched ahead of her.

VIRUS HACKER

When the process of viral infection is distilled to its most fundamental aspects, it resembles hacking: A virion enters a host cell by binding to a molecular lock on its surface. It carries a code in the form of a chemical signature that allows it to hack the lock. Once the connection is made, the virion downloads its genetic contents into the cell and reprograms it to generate copies of viral DNA. The cell then runs the viral program until it creates so many copies of the virus that it literally explodes.

Viruses, like hackers, take advantage of preexisting resources and reengineer them for their own selfish ends. Both crack and crash systems, disrupting the status quo, and in the face of that chaos they thrive. It would be difficult to come up with a more accurate parallel and yet it is a relatively recent one; to effectively peer into the behavior of viruses, networks and computers had to exist. Previous metaphors glossed over aspects of the infection process, or rather, they conceptualized viral action in a less meticulous way. An ancient, biochemical entity required, in a sense, the advent of technology to describe it. This produces a strange crackle in the mind; technology arises from a need, and then its products and processes are absorbed into culture as conceptual frameworks that then reorganize the world. The virus-hacker metaphor allows this mechanism to become visible. Beyond explaining viral behavior this situation reveals how we compose reality, which in turn reveals something else: the connection between the organic matter that makes us and what we ourselves make. This is why, perhaps, information is so susceptible to mutation online. Because we, ourselves, mutate constantly in response to our environment.

DESIGNATIONS

The word "Internet"—with a capital I—is used for the first time in 1982.

Also in 1982: the CDC gives the set of symptoms first identified in the June 5, 1981, *Morbidity and Mortality Weekly Report* a name: AIDS, or Acquired Immune Deficiency Syndrome.

NOIR IS A PLACE

Noir, at its crux, is about terrain. It is a genre about land, and how soil, sun, and shade give rise to atmosphere—both of the city and the soul. From this perspective, Los Angeles is the only city that could germinate this type of fiction, its sunny, arid conditions perfect to expose the shadows of the psyche. Of course, history books trace the origin to myriad cultural factors: postwar urbanization, the rise of consumer culture, moral decay, suburban expansion. They recall the migration of European filmmakers to Hollywood, fleeing fascism with nothing but the weight of German expressionism on their backs, but they leave out the fact that LA absorbed urban development *and* Fritz Lang. Los Angeles absorbed talent and situations and then spread itself through them. The city became embodied and it cycled through its citizens, and the citizens, immersed in the city, created new narratives around it, embedding the city in their creations, mythologizing it, formalizing it, and networking its many aspects together. As Bran Nicol writes in *The Private Eye: Detectives in the Movies,* "Noir might be thought of as a place in which whatever is 'black for us,' whatever troubles us, whatever we cannot resolve either in our personal lives or in our historical moment, is played out."

VIROLOGY 101

Lectures for a Virology 101 course at Columbia University are available for free on YouTube. The first lecture begins with the hotly debated question "Are viruses alive?" to which the impassioned professor quickly adds, "You can't know if viruses are alive if you don't know what life is."

IS THE INTERNET ALIVE?

In the years approaching 2020, the phrase "is the internet" would autocomplete to "alive" on Google. This meant a not insignificant portion of the population walked around wondering if the internet might have a mind of its own—assuming of course that by "alive" they meant "conscious."

The notion at first seems insane. Sure, the internet ruins lives, fixes lives, and creates and dissolves fortunes in the blink of an eye, but *alive*? The internet doesn't metabolize, have cells, or contain genetic material. Admittedly, however, it does possess equivalents, or metaphorical correspondences, to these life-defining traits. Following this logic, it is perhaps possible to imagine that these synthetic counterparts *could* give rise to something *like* life. That the hardware isn't biological material hardly seems to matter, at least according to neuroscientists subscribing to IIT, or integrated information theory, which posits "that consciousness arises from complex connections across different regions of the brain." From this perspective, consciousness is a by-product of interwoven relationships within a system rather than viscera. Christof Koch, proponent of IIT and head of the Allen Institute for Brain Science, explains,

> What matters is not the stuff the brain is made of, but the relationship of that stuff to each other. It's the fact that you have these neurons and they interact in very complicated ways. . . . If you could replicate that interaction, let's say in silicon on a computer, you would get the same phenomena, including consciousness. . . . The Internet now already has a couple of billion nodes. Each node is a computer. Each one of these computers contains a couple of billion transistors, so it is in principle possible that the complexity of the Internet is such that it feels like something to be conscious.

Essentially: the internet might have feels/be feeling itself/be in its feels, out of the dynamism of such sheer interconnectivity, but that doesn't mean it is "alive." This only places it in an indeterminate category of existence, not unlike the virus.

SOME DEFINITIONS OF CULTURE BY MERRIAM-WEBSTER

"The integrated pattern of human knowledge, belief, and behavior that depends upon the capacity for learning and transmitting knowledge to succeeding generations."

"Enlightenment and excellence of taste acquired by intellectual and aesthetic training."

"The act or process of cultivating living material (such as bacteria or viruses) in prepared nutrient media."

NOVEL RETROVIRUS

In 1983, a team of scientists at the Institut Pasteur led by Dr. Luc Montagnier isolates an unidentified retrovirus from lymph tissue belonging to a patient with lymphadenopathy, an opportunistic infection indicative of AIDS. The retrovirus is suspected to be an etiological agent of AIDS, and is named lymphadenopathy-associated virus, or LAV. These findings, published in the May 20 edition of *Science,* are groundbreaking; at present, there are only two other retroviruses known to infect humans, both of which have just recently been discovered by the American scientist Robert Gallo.

TIME IN A HOSPITAL

Time in a hospital moves differently than in other places. It is a substance you drift through, thick like water. The minutes and seconds submerge your body, weighing down the skin, dripping. The clock fused into the wall above the patient's doorway ticks too loudly. Its hands jerk forward reluctantly, like something out of a high school movie, but it kind of doesn't matter. You can't read the thing anyway. The whole apparatus falls apart, a series of lines and numbers that can barely contain themselves inside a circle. You realize how man-made it is. Time. The construct measures something completely different to what you are experiencing.

On the couch in Nivia's hospital room, time became a series of breaths. I stretched out on my back and focused all my senses on her respiration, as if I had a million tiny dials set into my pores that could be finely tuned to her precise frequency. I became an antenna receiving transmissions of inhalations and exhalations. Whenever even a hair of a variation in rhythm was detected, I'd launch myself off the couch straight to her bedside where I'd stare into her face, searching for the life still inside it, but the pauses were only ever brief anomalies, or figments of my imagination. By 5 A.M. I knew I wouldn't last much longer if I didn't permit my brain the distraction of at least one other sound, so I allowed myself the company of a single earbud and a podcast.

Very slowly I became aware of it, like a crack of light seeping in from under a door. I couldn't really make much of the voices. I had the sense they were forming something *like* words, but not words exactly. I left the episode on anyway.

It seemed to me that many years had passed in the last twenty-four hours. If I had had the courage to look out the window, I was convinced I'd see flying cars buzzing between wire-thin skyscrapers, or the gray powdered ash of a nuclear wasteland. My foot twitched and I whiplashed myself into a sitting position, gasping. As I dealt with the reverberations of this simple, involuntary motion, I began to understand I was listening to an episode of *Radiolab* about black boxes. I couldn't give a fuck, but then a strange thing happened: a single image rose up from some deep, undisclosed location, and floated into my thoughts. It was of sheets of newsprint gently fluttering in the breeze. They were clipped to a clothesline stretched over tiny desks. On them were drawings from my fifth-grade science class, scrawny lines of colored pencil and felt-tip marker depicting the black box concept. Trees, stars, airplanes, and sneakers entered funnels attached to opaque boxes, and emerged transformed on the other side as log cabins, fireworks, spaceships, and high heels.

I revolved these drawings and the faces of the kids who made them in my mind's eye, until something from the podcast crackled through: "My grandparents were mind readers on the radio." The words "grandparents" and "mind readers" shot through me like a bullet, and left a clean hole for the story to bleed into. Instantly, the tale of *The Piddingtons* absorbed me. The show, a live BBC radio production from the fifties, was based on the premise that Sydney and Lesley Piddington were an extraordinary couple, so extraordinary in fact that they shared a psychic bond. In its heyday, the estimated listenership was twenty million people. Each episode featured a "telepathy test" designed to highlight this supernatural connection. Oftentimes the tests were so extreme that the only plausible explanation for them was actual psychic activity. For heightened effect, the couple were always stationed in geographically disparate locations, with Sydney typically based in a West End theater, and Lesley somewhere mad like a diving bell at the bottom of the Thames, or in the Tower of London. To create another layer of bafflement, Lesley had to be cued to speak by technicians during broadcasts. She never wore headphones and so was never in direct contact with Sydney. Their act effectively was a black box. The audience could observe the setup of the test and the final result, but the telepathy itself was obscured.

Clips of *The Piddingtons* were patched throughout the *Radiolab* segment. The show's intro music resounded with the theatricality of a Hitchcock film, its organ conjuring a lonely mansion beneath a full moon. Under these ominous tones, Sydney's voice materializes, instructing the audience to remove numbered envelopes from beneath their seats. The combination of sonic elements makes it easy to picture him as a dapper gentleman, positioned at a "pill capsule" microphone encircled by a star. With a gentle charm, he asks everyone to write a few lines of text and seal it in their envelopes. He then selects two of these at random to "transmit" to Lesley, who, meanwhile, is in a plane soaring over Bristol. After some ceremony, the first envelope is opened and Lesley's voice appears. It flutters around in her throat, like a moth, delicately searching for the message vibrating through the ether. She finds something, an image, which begins to unfurl: "A bird . . . two birds . . ." The gauze of her consonants calls to mind Hollywood ingénues with their long, curled lashes resting atop doe eyes, and seemingly within a single bat of them, she unpacks the vision and sets it into a line of poetry: "Hail to thee, blithe spirit!" She sounds so breathlessly natural arriving at the correct answer, it's impossible not to believe her. The audience in the West End, bewildered, gasps and then applauds.

I heard something underneath the rustle of the audience's movement. A scratch from the recording equipment. I shifted my attention to focus exclusively on the white noise of the archival clips, and then I broke apart. I was listening to the world Nivia had lived in. I was listening to the time she existed in. I was *hearing* it, and I strained every nerve to catch the room tone, static, and clicks of those sound bites so I could be there with her. I set myself on fire, chasing every pop and glitch until, eventually, I lost them, and they blended into the rhythms of the medical devices measuring her heart rate and oxygen level. The sounds condensed back into one timeline, the one I was living in, and I pulled the earbud out. They were about to reveal the trick of the act, but I needed to remain in the dream of it. Besides, everyone knows things like this work through misdirection. All the clues are right there in front of your face, if only you are smart enough to see them.

Nivia made it through the night, and the next nine after that.

QUOTE FROM A TELEVISION SHOW

"What if it was really one long story that just kept
going and going until it healed itself? Wouldn't that
be a story worth telling? Wouldn't that be a story
worth hearing?"

—*True Detective*, "Now Am Found"

LA POLAROID

On my kitchen wall near the electric kettle is a mini-Polaroid of LA. A line of palm tree silhouettes cuts through the frame, and behind the blackened fronds, colors of a near-neon variety leak through the sky. The photo is held up by a strip of tape slowly weakening from daily interactions with kettle steam, and one of these days gravity will have its way with it. For the moment, though, the picture is holding, a long strand of hair trapped underneath the top right corner.

I keep the picture around to think of home. It allows things in my chest to circulate, but just briefly; the picture is small and so familiar to my eye I only catch it in distracted states, when my mind is splintered between so many tasks and places that the image can slip in uninvited.

THE SCREEN IS A MEMBRANE

Hacking is the primary metaphorical framework used to describe biological viral infection. The metaphor sets the biochemical entity within a technological space, casting host bodies as machines and viruses as subversive hackers. The inverse of this framework, or "going viral" in cyberspace, imbues the spread of information with biological connotations, for if a GIF or TikTok captures the internet, breaks it even, implicit in this spread is also the seizure of our organs. "Going viral" requires flesh, blood, and tissue for transmission. Information requires bones and brains, and we absorb it until it becomes part of us. We turn information into matter and exist through it. Cyberspace was once purely conceptual, but now what actually is the "space" of it? Where is the internet if not inside us? And perhaps this explains why people treat it as a living, breathing reality, creating multiple strands of existence on it. The screen is nothing more than a membrane. Stuff leaks in and out both ways.

In this respect, the virus's ascension into cyberspace seems less like a metaphor and more like the natural extension of its evolutionary trajectory. It mutates to survive, and, well, the hosts are online now, so—

DETECTIVE REPEATING GLANCE

I keep seeing an image of a detective with the brim of a trilby pulled low over the eyes and a trench coat collar flicked up, leaving only a sliver of face. This face looks at me, the one visible eye rotates slowly in its socket, traps me in its gaze, and then the whole figure turns away. It walks back into the shadows and leaves behind a cone of light striking a brick wall—and then, the scene rewinds. Black-and-white scan marks shred the image and pull it back on itself, as if all this were happening on VHS. The detective then reappears, casts a glance, and saunters into the darkness, only to reverse motion and resume the look, the loop on repeat scarred by glitching lines, almost to impress the point: the past is only past until you look at it again.

FLAG DAY

January 1, 1983, is heralded as "flag day" or the "birthday" of the internet. It marks the transition to a new communications protocol equivalent to a universal language; over the previous fifteen years, networks have proliferated globally and evolved in accordance with their own idiosyncrasies. Consequently, no standard form of communication exists for cross-network dispatches. The creation of the Transfer Control Protocol/Internet Protocol (TCP/IP) resolves this issue, enabling different types of computers across different types of networks to converse with one another. All future networks will be configured to these protocols.

METHODS OF VIRAL CULTIVATION

1. Live Animal Culture
   A living creature is used as a habitat to grow a virus.

2. Embryonated Egg Culture
   A virus is injected into a chicken egg and then incubated. The type of virus dictates its placement in the egg. For example: influenza is grown in the amniotic sac whereas the herpes simplex virus is placed in the chorioallantoic membrane.

3. Cell Culture
   Cells are grown in a nutrient-rich medium until they form a monolayer across their container, for instance, a petri dish. They are then injected with a sterilized sample of a virus and are placed into incubation for viral propagation of a noninfectious strain.

BLACKOUT

Vivian graduated from the Hunter College nursing program in 1966. A few months before receiving her diploma a severe power outage shrouded the island of Manhattan in total darkness. Hospitals in dire need of reinforcement reached out to the presumed graduates of medical programs across the city and drafted them as emergency support staff. Vivian and her three closest friends were called to Bellevue where, decked out in their starched caps and pristine white uniforms, they patrolled the halls of the psych ward, quietly, carrying open-flame candles.

RIP

Of course, if the internet is alive, it can also die.

"ON GRIEF OF MIND"

The first alleged nonagricultural use of the word "culture" occurred in the *Tusculanae Disputationes,* a text on Greek philosophy. Penned by Cicero around 45 B.C., it used the phrase "cultura animi" to suggest the psyche could be cultivated in the same manner as a grapevine: through strategic care and attention. He developed this concept during his withdrawal from public life. Tullia, his only daughter, had died after giving birth to her second son, and, overwhelmed by emotion, Cicero disappeared from Roman high society. He escaped to his villa in Tusculum, or more specifically: to its library, where he immersed himself in Greek classics. It was widely known that Tullia was his favorite child, and without her he wasn't sure how to exist. His only recourse was to study, searching for methodologies that would enable him to confront his pain. But, of course, he knew such an endeavor, even as he undertook it, was bound to fail. He wrote to his friend Atticus, "My sorrow defeats all consolation."

And yet, he worked. His many hours of library study evolved into the *Tusculanae Disputationes,* a text that delved into five different aspects of human experience. Their titles:

1. "On the contempt of death"
2. "On bearing pain"
3. "On grief of mind"
4. "On other perturbations of the mind"
5. "Whether virtue alone be sufficient for a happy life"

Tusculanae Disputationes is a work made from grief, about grief, that was also a distraction/remedy/aid for grief. Cicero was trying to write himself into another life, one without that mad, never-ending ache, and culture, or at least our conception of it as a collection or album of all human knowledge, stems from this, stems from a broken heart.

ANOTHER NOVEL RETROVIRUS?

In 1984, scientist Robert Gallo and a team of researchers at the National Institutes of Health isolate a novel retrovirus thought to be an etiological cause of AIDS. During the course of the year, Gallo will publish no fewer than four papers in *Science* that further solidify this conjecture. The virus is named HTLV-III as it is similar in character to Gallo's previous retrovirus discoveries of HTLV-I and HTLV-II.

HAND-HOLDING ICU

I reached outside of myself to the door, the hall, the stairs. I reached outside the building to where people stood smoking, talking to one another, but seemed generally vacant. I reached outside to a spot on the lawn where I thought I had dropped my rental car keys. They were there and I picked them up and I reached past the car, back to my airplane seat, and over the ocean, to another country, to another building, to the handle of another door, to my bed where my mind could rest while my body remained stationary, waiting. A doctor would be in soon to talk to me about Nivia's condition, but I didn't know when that would be so I sat stretching myself away and holding her hand.

Holding the hand of someone who is dying is difficult to explain because the grip of your own hand can fool you. The strength of it can jerk and echo through the hand that is leaving and, for a moment, you might mistake that for a response, a hello, when in truth, that hand is just becoming less dense. You can detect the retreat, the fade, the departure of the other through your own skin and so instinct makes you grip harder to maintain the feeling of pulse against pulse, to maintain the illusion of mutual pressure.

In this moment, every scene from every movie and TV show containing this hand-holding moment broadcast over my vision, and as I scrutinized all these moving pictures the words attached to them flooded my ears. The dialogue, peeled out of a thousand throats, entered my head, and my mind dispersed itself through it because I could not face where I was. An interference pattern of popular culture formed over my own feelings, confusing me and guiding me into a new reality.

Sitting in that chair, holding her hand, I could only feel I had been deposited into some overdetermined aspect of experience I would never be able to communicate because it would be arrogant, pathetic, or clichéd, and no sooner had such a self-indulgent thought crossed my mind than I felt my grandmother's hand slip out of mine and clock me across the jaw.

If only, I thought, over and over again, until my entire arm went numb.

CULTURE = LIFE CONTENT

If you have ever found yourself on the periphery, outside of dominant narratives and nuclear-ish families, you will have passed through a period of emptiness wherein the material of your life was not "suitable" for any of the things around you. Meaning: no outlet or form of communication existed to convey your experience, and so the experience remained caught inside you, seething. Without external channels to link to there's no way to transmit your information, so the internal landscape deactivates. It shuts down and remains inaccessible since no actions or language can scrape at it. Since you are, in fact, on your own.

The only recourse then is culture. Instead of one's experience, songs, podcasts, and TikToks are transformed into a shorthand for particular emotions or situations. At certain points in my life, if you asked me how I was I would have only been able to respond with data. I could summarize the latest *Game of Thrones* episode or recite the anecdote about Esther's dollar bill from *This American Life*. I could tell you about the *New Yorker* story of red honeybees and the "maraschino mogul," but I would not be able to answer even the simplest question about myself because I had nothing inside. I felt like a ghost and quite often when I entered a room I felt people pull away from me as if suddenly encountering a cold front. Maybe this fetishizes or romanticizes the situation, puts a metaphor on a state of being that quite possibly doesn't deserve one, but how do we talk about pain in a world full of pain? We can't. We don't even try. We talk about culture instead. That's why it spreads.

NOPE

Dr. Luc Montagnier's LAV and Dr. Robert Gallo's HTLV-III are proven to be the same virus in 1985. Naturally, a great controversy erupts: though Gallo was the first scientist to prove the causative relationship between the retrovirus and AIDS, word breaks out that the virus samples used for his studies actually came from Montagnier's lab. In addition, the Institut Pasteur files a patent dispute against the US Department of Health and Human Services regarding antibody tests for the virus. These legalities have an immediate trickle-down effect, delaying the creation and distribution of antibody tests urgently needed worldwide.

Perhaps on account of this dispute, President Ronald Reagan decides to publicly acknowledge AIDS for the first time.

DAPHNE ON INSTAGRAM

The other day on Instagram I saw a post by a Greek girl I used to work with. Daphne has a group of friends she's known since university. They holiday together. They picnic together. They watch Six Nations Rugby at West London pubs together. They are there when someone dies, gets married, has a baby, or an emergency appendectomy. During the workweek they make the effort to see one another despite whatever nonsense is going on. In the post, the six or seven of them all stand on separate steps of an escalator at the Tottenham Court Road tube station. Daphne's boyfriend, positioned on the lowest rung, takes the photo selfie-style of the whole gang behind him. They all bend in, cramming their upper bodies into frame, twisting into strange shapes to make sure all their faces can be seen. Despite the setup being cheesy as fuck the situation is somehow completely natural. Everyone is jubilant. The post would feel like a stab in the chest if it weren't so obviously taken on the fly. The spontaneity somehow keeps it genuine.

This scene is completely beyond my understanding. Maybe this kind of happiness only exists for certain people, in certain realities.

CYBERSTRATA

When something stops trending it is not stamped out or beaten down, but simply replaced. The old things, the worn-out things, silently fall to the ocean floor, drifting in slow motion through shafts of light. Once settled on the abyssal plain, they calcify and the process repeats. Information accumulates like mineral deposits, and through chemistry and pressure, crystalline bonds form between #thedress, Grumpy Cat, creepypastas, Keyboard Cat, the dancing baby, Baby Shark, Gangnam Style, lolcats, Friendster, #icebucketchallenge, the Harlem Shake, and #EdBallsDay. Our forgotten content builds up in layers of sediment and these layers contain our myths. They contain our distractions and vices. They contain our stories. In the future, people will read them and realize that we never once stopped to think about them.

LOOSE PHONE BOOK EQUIVALENT

The Domain Name System is implemented across the internet in 1985 to organize swarms of new hosts joining the digital landscape. The system assigns IP addresses to alphabetic hostnames, and then catalogs them via hierarchical categories, or domains, such as .com, .org, and .edu.

BASKING SHARK

The deeper you get into downtown Los Angeles, the more saturated your field of vision becomes with environmental detail, particularly after hours. The textures of brick, metal, and glazed sea-green tile slide over the eye. The recessed entryway of an old office building glows, its gold reliefs of chevrons and sunbursts burn like embers in the dark. In a shop window, mannequins wearing quinceañera dresses of taffeta and tulle float like jellyfish in an aquarium. Up on South Grand the metallic waves of Frank Gehry's concert hall freeze mid-crest, forever reveling in kinetic potential. Off Pershing Square an old life insurance office block done up in the Beaux-Arts style has decadent moldings of fruit, ribbon, and angel faces swelling and dripping down its cornices into even more extravagant scrolls and figures. One long, desolate block consists solely of jewelry stores, their display cases empty save for faded velvet cushions waiting to be of service. Then there are the old marquees, romantic and everywhere, some crumbling, some pristine, one with pink, green, and red neon tubes swirling into what once might have been fireworks. The Roxie Theatre still has its original sign, and its famous tiered roof still cuts a striking temple into the sky, though now it is a discount clothing store, one that throws its doors open during the day to expose its merchandise to the street. There are also "green spaces" with water features perpetually shut off due to some drought or another. On occasion, a lamppost left over from another era grows out of an intersection like an enchanted oak.

These elements provide a backdrop for a thousand dendritic narratives. They rustle around beautiful private school girls spilling out of greasy, unmarked bars, and homeless people silently pushing their shopping cart caravans through neglected plazas. They frame groups of men in flawlessly white T-shirts examining vintage cars, and lovers in hotel windows shimmying out of terry cloth robes. They harness these scenes into a single electric landscape of decay; in the late hours the peripheral emerges as the central action and the unconventional has the space to breathe. In these surroundings, in these moments, I do not feel abnormal but a part of the world, performing some essential function, such as an observer or recorder.

For a long time, I watched nighttime scenes play out as I drove. I drove odd hours because I was lonely, but when I was driving I didn't notice it because I wasn't in any one place or another, but moving between them in an undefined state of existence. When stationary, I was keenly aware of my heart having cracked open, rusting permanently ajar, aching to be of use . . . Now every once in a while, I catch a picture of a basking shark, a creature who spends the majority of its life with its jaws unhinged, and I think: yeah, that was in my chest. It still is. I know the beast is still there, but it no longer aggressively prowls in the way it once did. At least, for the time being.

SNEEZING

Sneezing is the body's method of coping with the inhalation of foreign matter. It is an involuntary reaction cultivated from millions of years of evolution to protect us from dust, allergens, and airborne contagions. Interestingly, the rhinovirus seems to have developed in concert with this defense mechanism. As Dorothy H. Crawford explains in *Viruses: A Very Short Introduction,*

The common cold virus (rhinovirus), while infecting cells lining the nasal cavities, tickles nerve endings to cause sneezing. During these "explosions," huge clouds of virus-carrying mucus droplets are forcefully ejected, then float in the air until inhaled by other susceptible hosts.

SEVERELY COMPROMISED

The retrovirus that causes AIDS is officially named "human immunodeficiency virus" in 1986. Naming the virus brings clarification to the HIV/AIDS constellation. According to the World Health Organization,

> Human immunodeficiency virus (HIV) is an infection that attacks the body's immune system, specifically the white blood cells called CD4 cells. HIV destroys these CD4 cells, weakening a person's immunity against infections such as tuberculosis (TB) and some cancers. If the person's CD4 cell count falls below 200, their immunity is severely compromised, leaving them more susceptible to infections. Someone with a CD4 count below 200 is described as having AIDS.

LEGEND OF THE PERPETUAL LAMP

Little is known of Tullia's life except for a few facts: whom she married and when they divorced, whom she married next, the names of her children, and her own nickname of Tulliola. The real details of how she moved across a room and what she longed for, her experience of color, were presumably never recorded, and if by some strange circumstance they were, time has evaporated them. The key to preserving what little of her remains is her parentage, her role as Cicero's daughter, and from that at least we know she was cherished.

But the story, strangely, does not end there. In the fifteenth century, Tullia's tomb was discovered. Accounts describe a nameplate declaring her identity, and a body so perfectly preserved it appeared as if she had only just been laid to rest. A dispatch from 1485 written by Daniele da San Sebastiano explains:

> In the course of excavations which were made on the Appian Way, to find stones and marbles, three marble tombs have been discovered during these last days, sunk twelve feet below the ground. One was of Terentia Tulliola, daughter of Cicero; the other had no epitaph. One of them contained a young girl, intact in all her members, covered from head to foot with a coating of aromatic paste, one inch thick. On the removal of this coating, which we believe to be composed of myrrh, frankincense, aloe, and other priceless drugs, a face appeared, so lovely, so pleasing, so attractive, that, although the girl had certainly been dead fifteen hundred years, she appeared to have been laid to rest that very day. The thick masses of hair, collected on the top of the head in the old style, seemed to have been combed then and there. The eyelids could be opened and shut.

According to the same account, flickering beside Tullia's body was a lamp, purportedly burning since her burial.

It's not important if any of this is true. The only thing that matters is that someone thought it should be true, as if Cicero's sorrow from all those years ago could be transformed into photons blazing across time.

ITCHY BRAIN

I sit at my desk with a beer bottle on it. The upstairs neighbor is doing laundry, the machine on spin cycle reverberates through my ceiling. The late afternoon light sinks into blue, and out on the street people are in transit, on their way to "going out." They are showered and fresh, sporting Converse sneakers and lightly applied eye shadow. They are in leather and denim, wearing Byredo perfume. The air crackles with the hope of lip-to-lip contact. Drinks are being had, cigarettes sizzle in the dark, desires are confessed. Life is aflame and burns into the weekend, but inside at my desk, I peel apart a single thought irritating my brain. There is nothing inside of it, save for a feeling: the pulsation of an acrylic fingernail tapping on a windowpane. A car stopped at the light on the corner blares "La Bamba." I take a swig of beer and then the engine fires and is gone.

AN AVERAGE GRAVE

In 1985, the NAMES Project AIDS Memorial Quilt is created by activist Cleve Jones in response to religious institutions and mortuaries refusing to host funerary services for AIDS victims. The Quilt, based in San Francisco, California, is a large-scale public arts initiative composed of fabric panels designed by people who have lost loved ones on account of the disease. Each panel measures three by six feet, or the size of an average grave.

SNOW WHITE

A friend in art school asked me about Nivia. I sighed, shook my head, and attempted to fold Nivia's life into a lucid narrative. When I finished, Amanda was silent for a while, and then began to systematically crush an empty beer can with one of her checkered Vans. In the aftermath of the gravel and aluminum scraping together she looked me in the eye and said, "Lady was a boss." I nodded and then we wordlessly headed back to our studios.

Nivia *was* a boss. A force field emanated from her tiny body that could elevate or shrivel whoever it came in contact with. The effects of this were mystifying, as most people could not figure out why a frail-looking, bitter, elderly woman should inspire total deference or fear in them. No one was immune. Even men who oozed a particular blend of machismo, such as plumbers and roof contractors, would become totally disarmed in her presence. This however was not a conscious deployment of charm or charisma on her part, or any other aspect of personality that could be employed for personal gain. It was simply a survival mechanism.

Nivia translates from Spanish to English as "Snow White," "Blanche Neige" in French, and drugstore hand lotion in a variety of different languages. She disliked her name, which was constantly mispronounced as Lydia, Livia, and Nidia. The situation was further exacerbated by her accent, as well as her choice to maintain her second husband's Scandinavian surname, which comprised a series of consonants strung together in a fashion deeply unfamiliar to the American eye. She also disliked direct sunlight, restaurant dining, pleasure of any nature, driving at night, department stores and their prices, cartoon animations, sweets, amusement parks, alcohol, cooking, and men, especially men—though she did love

Cary Grant. Grant's performance in *An Affair to Remember* raised a legitimate passion in her, as did a certain singer, except she could never remember the singer's name, or any of his albums. She referred to him only as "The singer I like, which one is he?" to which I'd say, "Luther Vandross? Julio Iglesias?" and sometimes, "Céline Dion?" in case she had mixed up her pronouns.

Nivia was born in 1923 in San Juan, Puerto Rico, to a mother who did not want or love her. She never knew the identity of her father, and the topic of her parentage was rarely discussed. The one or two times I witnessed it mentioned she attempted to kindly deflect for a few moments only to snap and bark out, "I was a bastard, okay!" The last of these outbursts occurred when she was eighty-six years old; despite the changing moral makeup of society and the many hours she spent in the company of Oprah, Ricki Lake, Montel Williams, and Sally Jessy Raphael, Nivia never got over the societal stigma tied to her origins. The shame of it haunted her until the day she died, as did the notion she had been born in the wrong era, and really, that she had been born at all.

The conditions of her upbringing were enough to shatter anyone's spirit, and Nivia had a clean fracture running down her psyche that in later years allowed her to house ideas and opinions that had no business inhabiting the same skull. To further add to this complexity, the split in her character would only reveal itself if she was prodded just so. Typically, she steeled herself within an armor of rationality, but if she felt herself threatened, even in the mildest regard, the armor would instantly evaporate and she would come at you with the tenacity of an old-school boxer, methodically clocking you in the face until you backed away, scuttling on all fours like the broken dog she told you that you were, and then, suddenly, the fever would leave her.

The contrast to this was a luminescence. Nivia had a love of learning so pure I have yet to come across it in another living soul. It held an otherworldly aspect I can only liken to characters in Dickens novels. Mathematically gifted, she had a piercing ability with figures and business, but was open to all forms of practical knowledge. This openness never abated. In her early eighties, she enrolled in piano and quilting courses at the Braille Institute in Los Angeles. The institute, twenty-five miles away, was only accessible to her via public transit. Her journey there involved three buses, one of which passed through the heart of South Central.

At age fourteen Nivia had to transfer to a middle school in a neighboring town, since her village schoolhouse ended at grade six. Prior to the start of the school year she traveled to the town and registered herself as a new student, also working out a free lunch scheme with the administration. The only remaining detail was the cost of daily transportation, which the school was unable to subsidize. With no other options she resigned herself to ask her mother for the bus fare, except she already knew the answer would be no. The reason for this was simply cruelty. Nivia would always tell me, "The bus was three cents a day. Three lousy cents my mother wouldn't give me!" And so, she went to work instead, becoming a seamstress.

Growing up I heard the three cents story many times, and with each retelling I felt myself grow dimmer. It was told in the same way that stories of this nature were deployed on family sitcoms pre-2000, where a visiting grandparent tells a sob story to remind the adolescent brat to stop acting like a nimrod: "When I was your age I walked ten miles, in the snow, without shoes . . ." On television it always did the trick, but the lesson seemed not to take offscreen. The hemispheres of my brain could not reconcile her life experience with my own, the material of our realities being so fundamentally different, and yet, the three cents story invaded me and lived underneath my mind along with the gesture she made while telling it: a flaring out of three fingers that resembled a peacock's tail.

Eventually Nivia escaped to New York City. I am unsure of the timeline, but she arrived with her young children and alcoholic husband in the 1940s. She sought work in the Garment District and found a position on a production line sewing dresses for department stores.

Initially, she was tasked with hand-stitching brand labels into the necks of dresses. She once explained to me that the high-end and midrange stores received the exact same dresses apart from this single detail. Consequently, she lost any respect she might have had for rich people. After her first shift, it became clear her skill level far exceeded the task, so she was instantly promoted. She spent a few weeks in various positions on the line until she was at the top, completing a full day's work before lunchtime. With half a day left to kill she found herself taking long "lunch breaks" that involved catching the matinee showing at Radio City. A friend, another girl with fast hands, often joined her, and when they returned to work, their manager, whom I always imagine as a balding, overweight, jolly fella in suspenders, would greet them, laughing, "So, girls, how was the picture?"

VIRAL VISIONS

Some facts about viruses:

1. "Viruses are the smallest of all microbes. They are said to be so small that 500 million rhinoviruses could fit on the head of a pin" (Microbiology Society).

2. "The oceans cover 65 percent of the globe's surface and, as there are up to 10 billion viruses per litre of sea water, the whole ocean contains around 4 x 10^{30} [viruses]—enough, when laid side by side, to span 10 million light years" (Crawford).

Thinking about sizes and quantities so foreign to our normal range of vision causes images to blossom across the mind's eye. The images arise from experience, or reels of "stock footage" subconsciously hoarded over the years. Facts are consumed and visualizations effortlessly unspool to ground what is completely beyond our typical frames of reference.

In the case of these two examples, however, the mental reflex fails. These bits of knowledge only succeed in highlighting our physical limitations: no naked eye will ever see five hundred million viruses, but a pin is familiar; to get my head around the quantity of viruses in the ocean, I must reach out into space, far beyond the observable universe:

GOOGLE DEATH

I let the internet show me its late-night thoughts on death. The glow of the screen burns into my face. My skin catches hold of it and projects it back into the darkness of the room. For a split second, I am like the moon, nothing but a reflective surface. I forget I have a body and then I dissolve completely into GIFs of vintage skeleton cartoons, silhouettes of the Grim Reaper, coffins, ravens, the hooded figure from *The Seventh Seal,* ischemic heart disease, chronic obstructive pulmonary disease, and questions like: Why do people die? What is the first sense to go when you are dying? How

to identify a body? Does dying hurt? I diffuse through definitions—
"Death is the permanent cessation of all biological functions that
sustain a living, physical organism," "Death is the permanent ending of vital processes in a cell or tissue," "the state of being dead"—
and listicles:

Lists of Unusual Deaths

Unusual Deaths Throughout History

Freaky Deaths: 19 Bizarre Ways That People Have Kicked the
Bucket

32 Incredibly Weird Deaths That Will Make You Glad to Be Alive

13 Celebrity Deaths That Were Just Bizarre

I click on this last one and learn that the Crocodile Hunter was not,
as I had assumed, mauled to death by a giant, semi-aquatic reptile,
but killed by a stingray, a jab straight to the heart.

On Wikipedia, Death's entry has a collection of rather poetic
images interspersed between the usual diagrams and color-coded
graphs. At the top of the page is a close-up of a skull missing its
front teeth. It looks prehistoric, more reminiscent of a Neanderthal
than you or me, or alas, poor Yorick, and just below is a photo of an
anatomically detailed skeleton statue carrying a scythe. A delicate
shroud billows around its spine as one of its hands meagerly points
forward. Next comes the image of a limp Eurasian magpie, its body
an oily hunk of iridescent feathers. Scrolling down, a seventeenth-
century painting composed of dark shadows clinically displays a
variegated tulip, a bronze skull (also curiously short of teeth), and
an inauspicious hourglass on a slab of gray stone. A memento mori,

but also a hyperlink to the entries on Life and Time. I abandon ship and return to Google, feverishly typing in as many permutations of death as I can think of: loss, loss of loved one, dead relative, dead parents, grief, aggrieved, mourning, mourner, melancholy, heartbreak, void . . .

I click on every single link I come across, until I can no longer tell what I'm looking at, but, eventually, through the glowing blur I land on something that might prove useful, an essay in *Slate* titled "Finding a Metaphor for Your Loss." The author writes of her mother's death and the strange paradox of not feeling her depart. She simply felt her mother "transferred into another substance," specifically the wind. The wind became the metaphor for her loss.

I close the clamshell of my laptop with a grain of something. I have no sense my parents are dead. I simply have no sense of anything at all. What might the metaphor for that be?

SETTLEMENT

American President Ronald Reagan and French Prime Minister Jacques Chirac end the patent dispute regarding the HIV antibody tests in 1987. An agreement is forged stating both nations will share the royalties of the patent, and the scientific prestige of the discovery, equally.

WHY WE TALK ABOUT IT

In a *Los Angeles Review of Books* essay, Elizabeth Winkler writes, "The strategic logic of the 21st century is the logic of the virus. . . . Contagion is, in fact, the condition to which all politicians, business owners, and entertainers aspire."

Humans adopting the sensibility of a virus for commercial or financial domination hints at a buried nature, of something crawling forth from the primordial ooze, and perhaps a mechanism etched out in our DNA is in fact bubbling to the surface. The question is: Why? Why did we start talking about ideas, or a person's face, going viral? Winkler goes on: "We talk about virality not just because the world is interconnected or overpopulated; we talk about it—or, at least, we first talked about it—because of HIV."

NURSE'S CAP

The square box is faded now, but it must have once been a brilliant shade of sky blue, the tonal equivalent of quotidian pink-pastry bakery boxes. Inside, wrapped in a single sheet of brittle tissue paper, is Vivian's nurse's cap. The shape is nearly indescribable, a comedic hybrid of a housemaid's headpiece from a period drama and a flying saucer—the thing is starched to the high heavens. It will never lose its form, just like an arrowhead flint sheathed in ash.

RESURRECTION

AZT, the failed anticancer drug of the sixties, is resurrected during the US nationwide search for medicines that might prove effective in the treatment of HIV/AIDS. Clinical trials have shown evidence that AZT facilitates weight gain in patients with AIDS and assists with the restoration of T cell immunity. Facing pressure from activists in addition to the growing epidemic, the Food and Drug Administration accelerates the approval of the drug. This is not without controversy: not only are the long-term effects of the drug unknown, but many physicians believe the potential toxicity of AZT might kill patients faster than HIV itself.

BLACK HOLE

Without someone or something to anchor you to the world, holes form in your brain. At times the gravitational force of these holes will become so powerful your life will get pulled directly into them, but to fall into a cavity that is inside of you, to be swallowed through from the inside—isn't that like being consumed by a black hole? Isn't that the definition of noir? To be sucked down into a place where not even light can escape?

SIGH

Of course, if people want to think the internet is alive there's no stopping them.

ALCHEMY

What is it to remember a photograph instead of the real thing? To know a picture by heart so well and to recall it accidentally as fact, is this really so different from remembering the flesh-and-bone event that also unfolded in image after image after image? Of course it is different, except not nearly as much as we want it to be, or think it should be, because memory is an invention in the same vein as Instagram or the video camera and we understand it now primarily in relation to all the devices we have built to emulate it. What did memory look like before photography? No one knows. No one remembers. No one is alive to tell us what recollections looked like before we had things that could freeze time and pre-serve its remnants.

I imagine that, for the generation who lived through the emergence of photography, remembering a photograph instead of the actual event must have seared through the skull, and for those who came later, raised with snapshots and vacation slides, I imagine the mistake felt more like a glitch, or a hiccup, than a burn. But now, to hold a picture so dear you make it real? To love it so much it acquires skin and grows a past and walks around, what is the sensation of this new reality? Of two dimensions becoming three? What does it *actually* feel like? How do we speak of this new twist of evolution? And, on the other hand: What is it to make a moment tangible, to cut it out from life, disengage it from the present and materialize it in kilobytes? Isn't this alchemy?

CRASHING, OR INCREASED NUMBERS

In 1988, the Morris worm is unleashed by Robert Tappan Morris, a graduate student at Cornell University. Conceptualized as a tool to scout the size of the internet, the worm is accidentally destructive, crashing every system it comes in contact with. This results in a quarantine of 10 percent of the world's internet servers. With damage so widespread, Morris becomes the first person tried and convicted under the Computer Fraud and Abuse Act of 1986. Years later he will become a tenured professor at MIT, possibly due to the fact that his worm, aside from the damage, was something of a landmark: it was the first to move through the internet via weaknesses in network applications. Meaning: no hardware required.

In 1989, the CDC reports 100,000 cases of AIDS in the US.

DAD ASHES

We kept Vivian's makeup for a long time after she died, almost twenty years. It was the makeup she used for work, the understated yet elegant shades for contouring and the instruments she used to apply them. A white plastic case with silver logo lettering contained a trio of blushes, and another identical case held eye shadows in plum, midnight, and sand dune. A circular pad of the kind used in mirrored compacts had decades' worth of foundation soaked into it. Eroded bits of its sponge broke off from time to time and left a crumb trail between blunt kohl eyeliner pencils and brushes with imitation mother-of-pearl handles. These objects, in addition to an eyelash curler and a bottle of YSL Paris perfume, were kept in a linen basket that emitted the scent of a department-store cosmetics section.

Nivia preserved this trove because she believed items of utility had a second, third, or even fourth life. Her rationale was that I would eventually "inherit" these products, completely oblivious to the fact that they, like people, were subject to decay. At the same time, I was forbidden to wear makeup, which made her hoarding all the more peculiar. Determined to keep me cryogenically frozen as a child, she delayed, or rather attempted to delay, my exposure to certain life experiences, of which eyeliner was one. Fortunately, I had no real interest in makeup. I bought my first lipstick when I was twenty-eight.

Over the years the blushes and powders disintegrated. They crumbled, became chalk, and vaporized, particle after particle. This was what I had left of my mother. Not her library. Not her cassette tapes. Not her silk scarves, nor the brooches she used to keep them gently pinned across her neck. Not her framed lithographs of Jupiter or Orion, but a desiccated mascara wand with broken bristles like fish bones. The possessions I might have been able to look at later in life and examine with an archaeologist's eye were simply gone. For a while I managed to hold on to her address book, which contained lines that actually came out of her hand. The curves and marks of it were preserved in the names and numbers of the people she knew, and maybe even loved. The book itself was an album of her floral capitals. I could have made it a fixture of my daily reality, but I stowed it at the back of a desk drawer, psychically cherishing its faux-leather cover with brass accents. One day, of course, it vanished too.

My father, David, by contrast, had very few personal effects, so their erasure felt more like math; one day his prescription glasses and his wristwatch were there, the next day they were not. A simple, observable subtraction. The stapler from his desk set, however, was retained. Nivia perceived its use and adopted it as her own. After her death, while clearing out her office belongings, I found it, a Bates model 640. I held the metal two-tone design in my hands, and crumpled to the floor. Of all things to survive, his stapler? I choked, laughing, but I understood. The stapler had a distinct function, whereas his glasses did not, nor his remains. After David was cremated, Vivian kept his ashes in the trunk of her Subaru. She liked the idea they were still "on the road together," but then she became too weak to drive, and the car was sold. And the ashes? Who knows. For a long time his death overshadowed everything else. The notion of his final resting place seemed so trivial compared to the fact that he was no longer on Earth, but then, ever so slowly, it started to seep into my mind, one small layer at a time, that this might be unusual. I mean, it's weird not to know where your dad is buried, right?

ELECTRON MICROSCOPE

No one saw a virus until 1939. Too small to be read by even the strongest of light microscopes, viruses remained speculative until technology evolved to confirm their existence.

The invention that would eventually image them, the electron microscope, was developed in Berlin in 1933. The physicist Ernst Ruska and electrical engineer Max Knoll created the first model, riffing on the design of the popular compound microscope. For their device, Ruska and Knoll swapped out traditional convex glass lenses for coiled electromagnets, and added a laser beam of charged electrons that, when fired through a specimen, could gather detailed information about its structure. As electrons have much smaller wavelengths than photons, specimens of minute sizes could now easily be imaged.

However, in 1933, virtually no one cared about submicroscopic vision, particularly in Germany. Investors regarded the endeavor as a vanity project with no widespread industrial application. Dejected, Ruska was ready to can the whole enterprise when his brother intervened. Helmut Ruska, a man of the biological sciences, immediately understood the wondrous value of the instrument and believed it could revive research in several scientific disciplines that had languished precisely due to the lack of powerful imaging technology. The benefit to medicine alone would be colossal, so Helmut reached out to his former mentor at the renowned Charité hospital and asked him to endorse the device. The success of the electron microscope boils down entirely to this link between personal histories and disciplines. Six years later, the first electron micrographs of TMV were published and made available to the scientific community.

A webpage dedicated to Helmut states, "The visualisation of virus particles brought reality to the theoretical concepts in virology and thus, led to a thorough understanding of an entirely new world of pathogens."

Somehow it always comes down to seeing is believing.

PHONE SEX?

Working the graveyard shift on the seventeenth floor of a Parisian high-rise, the guy goes about his tasks in the dark. He leaves the fluorescent overheads off, wanting the mist of the city's illuminations to radiate upward and fill his visual field. Apart from his typing, everything is quiet, the building doesn't even hum. On occasion, one of the wheels of his swivel chair squeaks as he shifts back and forth between Minitel terminals. His night consists of this dance between machines; each one is logged in to a different sex chat room, and he operates in all of them, as different women. He rotates through a catalog of personas, the most crowd-pleasing of which is a "nineteen-year-old bisexual student." People naturally tell her their fantasies, but oddly, just as naturally, they tell her about their lives and the fears within them. For around a dollar a minute they peel themselves open like tangerines, and let their brilliant torn rinds fall in clumps by the wayside.

The guy is unaccustomed to this vulnerability. There is no room for it, for the tender pith of a person, during waking life, so he has never before had to face it, but at night, behind the screen, something happens. The technology has brought with it a new dimension; through the wires, space uncoils. Emotions become frictionless, and they seamlessly glide as glowing boxes of text down a sheet of glass.

Years later, on a podcast, the guy will admit that all of this changed him. As a person. He will remark that every morning when he left the office, he'd stumble into a stream of zombie-like commuters and wonder how many of them he had spoken to just hours before. He will say that, somehow, this made him a writer.

CIRCLES AND ARROWS

At the end of the eighties, Tim Berners-Lee, an independent contractor at CERN, conceptualizes the World Wide Web in a proposal written out of frustration. Troubled by work inefficiencies created by information mismanagement he outlines a "hypertext database with typed links" that could sit on top of the internet as an application. He suggests that the intuitive, everyday communication style between CERN employees should be replicated in this database. Berners-Lee writes:

> CERN is a wonderful organization. It involves several thousand people, many of them very creative, all working toward common goals. Although they are nominally organized into a hierarchical management structure, this does not constrain the way people will communicate, and share information, equipment and software across groups.
>
> The actual observed working structure of the organization is a multiply connected "web" whose interconnections evolve with time. . . . The hope would be to allow a pool of information to develop which could grow and evolve with the organi-

zation and the projects it describes. For this to be possible, the method of storage must not place its own restraints on the information. This is why a "web" of notes with links (like references) between them is far more useful than a fixed hierarchical system. When describing a complex system, many people resort to diagrams with circles and arrows. Circles and arrows leave one free to describe the interrelationships between things in a way that tables, for example, do not. The system we need is like a diagram of circles and arrows, where circles and arrows can stand for anything.

MARLOWE KNIGHT

The detective genre is built solely on perception and observation. As Bran Nicol writes in his treatise on the private eye in cinema, "We see what the detective sees, usually when and how he sees it. Prose fiction offers an equivalent experience: the first-person perspective favoured by the hard-boiled novel means its world is always filtered through the consciousness of the detective-narrator; we never inhabit it 'objectively.'"

The scenes I observed during my adolescent late-night drives resembled ones I read about years later in novels by Raymond Chandler. The gaze that described Los Angeles in those books was eerily similar to the one I employed to view my surroundings. The overlap of vision struck something lodged in my core; I found myself pulled to Chandler's detective, Philip Marlowe.

Detectives tell us stories that are not their own. Their cases substitute their own personal history. There is no before and after with them, just an unfolding of episodes. What Marlowe fixates on might be the echo of a previous experience reverberating through him, but the original event is inaccessible to us, locked in a shell of oxidized metal, or perhaps: a rusty suit of armor. One perspective of noir regards the detective as the genetic descendant of heroes from the Romantic tradition, such as Arthurian knights. This prospect is less far-fetched than it sounds when considering that both genres revolve around a quest; like the knight, the detective is on a quest for truth, but the detective inhabits a morally ambiguous universe. In Arthurian legends, truth is absolute, and it does not get the knight's nose busted in or sliced open when he discovers it. Quite the contrary, the knight's adherence to a code—chivalry—ensures his protection, whereas the detective's obsession with maintaining a strict moral code inevitably results in a body count. Marlowe's anachronistic sense of right and wrong is a direct inheritance from Sir Galahad but has no place in postwar Los Angeles. The city, in fact, gnaws away at it, like acid, though Marlowe holds steadfast, which suggests that he himself is a romantic. He lets it slide out in thoughts like: "No feelings at all was exactly right. I was as hollow and empty as the spaces between the stars."

Underneath the rusted armor is a pulse, a lonely one, and . . . I love him. I love him *and* I want to be him. Always on the verge of giving up, Marlowe never actually caves. Instead, he focuses on investigation; he uses his cognitive capacities to resolve disturbances in society. Instead, he drinks. He uses words sparingly, and then throws them like darts. The impulse to keep going, to survive, is something I recognize, and I often wonder about a character cut from the same moth-eaten cloth, possessing the same attributes and disposition, but modernized, and: a woman. What does it look like when she roams the streets? Drives down the coast? Gets smacked around by the cops because she won't sell out a friend? What does it look like when she watches life from a diner window or through the dusty venetian blinds of her office? A detective, after all, is just an eye. It is a profession, Nicol writes, "figuratively reduced 'to the organ of visual perception,'" which means these stories are really about nerve—and I need to see this nerve wired into a woman. I need to see if I could be anything like her.

TRANSATLANTIC RELATIONS

"When I first heard of the electron microscope which was said to have been developed in Germany, it almost seemed to be a hoax perpetrated on the rest of the world by the Nazis. It should be recalled that in 1940 our relations with Germany were so strained that it was difficult to obtain current literature from that country."

— THOMAS F. ANDERSON, American biophysicist

BACKBONE

ARPANET is decommissioned in 1990 and replaced by the National Science Foundation Network—NSFNET—which only services governmental and academic institutions. As more institutions become networked, NSFNET grows in complexity and geographic reach until it is deemed a "backbone" of the internet. The internet of today is an outgrowth of this spine.

METAPHORS WE THINK WITH

In 2011, the Department of Psychology at Stanford University released a study titled "Metaphors We Think With: The Role of Metaphor in Reasoning." The researchers sought to investigate the possible correlation between the language we use to discuss ideas and the mental framework we use to construct them. In other words, are metaphors "just fancy ways of talking, or do they have real consequences for how people reason?" To more thoroughly examine the question, it was contextualized within the discourse of social issues, specifically crime. The objective was to empirically determine whether "we reason about complex social issues in the same way that we talk about them: through a patchwork of metaphors."

Crime discourse overflows with metaphors, and, combing through a variety of textual material ranging from academic essays to eyewitness accounts, the researchers selected the two most popular yet diametrically opposed metaphorical frameworks to work with. Five experiments were designed using these frameworks, each testing for the potential of metaphors to influence reason.

In the first experiment, participants were asked to read a paragraph of text and then respond to a series of follow-up questions. Half of the participants read:

> Crime is a wild beast preying on the city of Addison. The crime rate in the once peaceful city has steadily increased over the past three years. In fact, these days it seems that crime is lurking in every neighborhood. In 2004, 46,177 crimes were reported compared to more than 55,000 reported in 2007. The rise in violent crime is particularly alarming. In 2004, there were 330 murders in the city, in 2007, there were over 500.

The other half read:

> Crime is a virus infecting the city of Addison. The crime rate in the once peaceful city has steadily increased over the past

three years. In fact, these days it seems that crime is plaguing every neighborhood. In 2004 . . .

Both sets of readers were then asked to provide methods for dealing with Addison's crime problem. The crime-as-beast readers suggested proactive and aggressive measures to curtail the threat, such as "catching and jailing criminals and enacting harsher enforcement laws," while the crime-as-virus readers proposed more strategic solutions, like "investigating the root causes and treating the problem by enacting social reform to inoculate the community." Each group consistently proposed solutions in line with the framework they were exposed to. This data, coupled with results from the other four experiments, confirmed that metaphor plays a role in reasoning about social issues.

The takeaway is that once an issue is framed for us we interface with it primarily on those terms. We maintain the integrity of the idea and create content or opinions *in harmony with it*. Strangely, we are oblivious to this. Another follow-up question asked participants to highlight aspects of the report that were "most influential" in leading them to their proposed solutions. Without fail, the participants underlined the statistical data as backup for their opinions and completely overlooked the metaphorical language. Metaphors, it seems, have the capacity to infect our thought process and incubate in our minds, undetected. We are as susceptible to them as we are to contagion.

HOW I THINK YOU BECOME A PERSON

You absorb a thing and then you do a thing, then you absorb that thing to do another thing, and then all these things become intertwined until heat and pressure congeal them into a sequence in your mind. The process repeats. The sequences accumulate, mingle, and interlock to form a history that can be shared, and it is through such exchanges that you realize, against all odds, you've become a person.

AIRPLANE GIRL

I don't know much about my father. I don't like to talk about it because there are already so many stories of missing fathers, and awful, poisonous, lunatic fathers, fathers who murdered and fathers who lied, fathers who left, ran, hit, touched, fathers who swindled, and fathers who drank, that I don't feel quite right adding my own story, which is only of a dead father, to that particular river of sorrow. In truth, I have managed okay without him, and I am only bothered by his death on rare occasions. He died before I had any adult grasp of his character, so in a sense there is little to recall. I was seven when he died, barely cognizant of anything beyond my own nose let alone the intricacies of personhood. More so, he was terminally ill for at least the last year of his life, confined to a hospital bed in his office and basically hidden from me.

The last time he genuinely crossed my mind was about two years ago on a Virgin Atlantic flight from Los Angeles to London. Shortly after takeoff, I noticed a father and teenage daughter sitting a few rows behind me on the window side of the aircraft. During the flight, they hardly exchanged a word. The father would ask a question and the daughter would respond with a grunt or a sigh. When we touched down at Heathrow and the seat belt sign chimed throughout the cabin, the father began chitchatting with another passenger, a classic English gent type, clearly a banker. As the father protectively maneuvered his girth into the aisle he explained he was in town for business but had brought his daughter along as an early high school graduation present. He took a deep breath before reaching down to extract his polished briefcase from under his seat and when he was vertical again his face carried a deep blush inside it.

Slightly out of breath, he managed to rattle off their itinerary: tea at Claridge's, the V&A, a ride in an open-topped double-decker bus for a general view of the city. The English passenger said this sounded like a marvelous introduction to London indeed and asked where they were staying. "The Connaught," the father replied, at which point I stopped listening.

I turned my attention to the daughter wedged in at a right angle in her seat row. Her face was a mixture of irritation and boredom, but I couldn't make out much more than that. She was average in every respect: not pretty, not unattractive, not tall, not short, not blond, not brunette, just a muted blur of a human, and while blending in to one's surroundings is common, on closer inspection most people have something detectable going on beneath the skin—an intelligence, a curiosity, a warmth. You can feel, in short, a mind at work, but there was no hint of any synaptic activity occurring in this girl's skull. All she had was the air of someone never forced to distinguish herself to the outside world. I watched her reach for her expensive yet completely tasteless leather bag from the overhead compartment, and her arm swung upward as if completely severed from her consciousness. The nature of the movement so profoundly disturbed me that when she whipped around and snapped, "Dad!" I trembled. I can only assume I missed a line of "dad humor" as the two men shared a laugh that concluded with the word "Kids!" and a shrug.

Grabbing my bag and coat I understood that one day this girl's life would be disrupted by her father's death, but in no way upended. Her existence already neatly fit into a prescribed narrative, and this privilege would serve as a shield against the dark night of the soul. In fact, she could probably go her entire life without a soul.

I stayed in my seat for much longer than was necessary. I wanted to make sure they were well off the plane before I disembarked. All I could think was: this girl has everything and has no fucking idea, and somewhere in that, my father appeared.

THEORIES OF VIRAL EVOLUTION

- The "virus-first hypothesis" suggests viruses predate all cellular organisms, and possibly had a role in their creation. It is thought their emergence as the first self-replicating entities may have precipitated the development of all other life forms.

- The "regressive hypothesis" suggests viruses "regressed" from cellular organisms, and thus are a by-product of them.

- The "escape hypothesis" suggests viruses emerged from "escaped" fragments of genetic material associated with cellular organisms, and thus evolved concurrently with them.

RED RIBBON

Visual AIDS, a New York–based organization that "utilizes art to fight AIDS," creates the red ribbon symbol in 1991. It is adopted worldwide as a symbol for HIV/AIDS consciousness and compassion.

SIGHT

Sight is the process by which light enters the eye and creates an image in the brain. Eons of evolution have fine-tuned the structures of the human eye to more effectively control the focusing of light toward the optic nerve; the cornea, lens, and pupil all work in concert, adjusting themselves by thickening, dilating, or bending to guide photons directly to the retina. Of all the tissues in the body, the retina might be the most unusual. It lines the very back of the eye like a half shell, but it is more than just insulation:

> The eye is formed during embryonic development by a combination of head ectoderm and neural tube tissue, the latter forming the retina. Thus, the retina is not a peripheral sensory organ like skin touch receptors or taste buds on the tongue, but rather it is an outgrowth of central nervous tissue. Because of this origin, the retina has layers of neurons, internal circuits, and transmitters characteristic of the brain: it is a bit of the brain that has journeyed out, literally, to have a look at the environment.

The retina unfurls from the brain like a tendril. Its specialized photoreceptor cells break an image apart, separating it out into color and brightness. These respective datasets are then translated into electrochemical signals that are read by other cells. These turn into nerve impulses that cascade down the optic nerve, spilling eventually into the occipital lobe.

How light becomes electricity or chemistry inside the body to form pictures baffles me. Not the science of it, which can be explained through proteins and shape-shifting membranes, but the possibility of such a thing happening in the first place. How do electrical signals produce, say, *L'Avventura*? That Antonioni's film can be parsed and translated into the language of cells and decoded as a series of black-and-white moving images within a loose narrative seems outrageous, and yet there is perhaps nothing more mundane than seeing an image and grasping its contents. The systems of the eye are so fragile that glitches are inevitable, and yet the process of sight appears to *consistently* give us a one-to-one correspondence with our surroundings.

In other words: how does a nerve impulse give rise to experience?

CHAMELEON VIRUS

In March 2014, Mashable UK ran a story about the Chameleon virus, a piece of malware created by researchers at the University of Liverpool. The virus was designed to mimic airborne contagion and spread through hosts "like a cold." To hammer home the point, the article was paired with an evocative black-and-white photograph that triggered an immediate visceral recoil, as if you might catch something by looking at it.

Taken in close-up, the photograph features a man sneezing in profile. The use of a high-speed camera has enabled the preservation of every micro-muscular movement and snot globule in pristine detail. The fat of his face is smooshed backward, his lips are unnaturally peeled apart. A dramatic arc of vapor erupts from his

flared nostrils, and against the black of the background the moisture appears like a million glistening stars. Were it not for the face
and description, we might temporarily forget about the mucus, but
the caption reads, "Photograph shows spray droplets from the
mouth and nose at velocities of up to 150 feet per second."

The image and content of the article cross-contaminate and suddenly the prospect of a computer virus circulating through the atmosphere becomes absolutely chilling.

The Chameleon virus works by hovering in the background of
Wi-Fi networks and searching for weak points where devices con-
nect to the internet. Rather than infect the actual devices, the virus
contaminates these access points and hops between them, using
them effectively as gateways to different networks. As it spreads, it
collects data on user behavior, data that of course can be sold,
mined, or monetized for nefarious purposes. Antiviral software
leader McAfee writes on its blog, "And, as with a cold, the success
of this virus depends on population density. The more Wi-Fi networks with overlapping access points, the more likely an infection
will occur and more likely the virus will spread." While classical
malware aims to destroy networks, the purpose of Chameleon is
simply to blend in and observe, as if it were part of the scenery.

TRUE DETECTIVE

The TV show is about two detectives and their relationship. It
moves between three timelines: the distant past, when the detectives are young, cocky, and just starting out, the more recent past,
in which the detectives are still cocky but jaded, and the present, in
which the detectives are no longer cocky but are old men worn

down by the wheel of the world. In each of these timelines the same case is addressed: the disappearance of two children, a brother and sister, seemingly into thin air. This lack of evidence does not sit well with these guys, so they heroically persevere until they uncover some leads. However, every time the case is on the verge of closing, a loose thread emerges that drags it into the future. In one timeline, the body of the boy is found. In another, a phone-line tip suggests the girl is still alive, but where? This lingering question is most poignant in the present-tense timeline, as one of the detectives develops a sickening suspicion that the key to the case is *finally* right in front of him, but he just can't seem to see it. He is unsure whether this is because a tiny shred of evidence might be misplaced, or if he's just losing his mind; he has Alzheimer's and therefore good days and bad days, and others where his neurons malfunction and the lines between past and present break down and comingle. He has visions. Hallucinatory? Celestial? Symptomatic? We don't know. You can read it any which way, but while his memory goes, his detective instincts remain intact and eight episodes in he does solve the case, he does find the girl, but we know he won't remember. The "truth" of what happened will be lost, like everything else, to time.

The epiphany comes in a mesmerizing scene: he picks up a book written by his late wife, which recounts the unsolved case in great detail, and in a synaptic explosion, he puts together the events of the recent days with a few sentences he's peeled off the page and he realizes he's found the girl! He's met her face-to-face, and then suddenly his wife appears. She whispers in his ear, "All this life, all this loss. What if it was really one long story that just kept going and going until it healed itself? Wouldn't that be a story worth telling? Wouldn't that be a story worth hearing?"

UPDATES

On April 30, 1993, CERN releases the World Wide Web to the public for free.

In November, statistics listed in the *Morbidity and Mortality Weekly Report* confirm HIV disproportionately affects marginalized communities:

> Stratified by race, HIV infection was the leading cause of death for black men aged 25–44 years during 1991 and 1992 (21.4% and 25.3% of deaths, respectively) and the second leading cause of death (preceded by unintentional injuries) for white men in that age group (17.8% in 1991 and 18.5% in 1992). HIV infection was the second leading cause of death for black women aged 25–44 years (up from third in 1991) in 1992 (12.1% in 1991 and 16.5% in 1992) and the sixth leading cause of death for white women aged 25–44 years in 1991 and 1992 (3.4% in 1991 and 3.8% in 1992).

In August of the following year, the White House establishes a web presence, whitehouse.gov.

SOME EXAMPLES

> "Highways, webs, clouds, matrices, frontiers, railroads, tidal waves, libraries, shopping malls, and village squares are all examples of metaphors that have been used in discussions of the Internet."
>
> — Wikipedia

ARCHITECT

There are periods when I think about Vivian's first husband more than I think about her. He was an acclaimed architect based in Malibu and had designed their home, which hovered above the Pacific Ocean on stilts. The water would sweep under the living room and would make you feel like a deity floating over the waves. I knew about the house and his profession solely through Nivia, both of which she brought up a few times to say something to the effect of "Your mother could have lived like a movie star and instead married your father." But once she went further with the architect: "If he ever saw you his heart would stop."

"Why?"

"Because you look exactly like your mother."

"Does he know she's dead?"

She avoided answering me.

After Nivia died, I found in her records a document linking Vivian and the Architect. I immediately googled him. The first hit was his obituary, which, for reasons I can't fully explain, devastated me. Aside from a list of professional achievements a mile long, it mentioned he had been "happily married" for thirty-six years and father to two sons. He was also a "Porsche aficionado." This agitated something in my mind, and dim memories of my mother's Porsche rose to the surface. She sold it when I was three, and I could feel in her something ending, though I was at a loss for what it was or what it might mean. All I knew was that it seemed like more than a car was driving away from us when the new owner came to collect it.

TRIPLE COCKTAIL

In 1995, the FDA approves a new type of antiretroviral drug that proves pivotal in the treatment of HIV. Saquinavir, a protease inhibitor, works by forcibly binding to HIV viral enzymes (proteases) and blocking (or "inhibiting") their function during viral replication. The introduction of saquinavir to HIV management paves the way for HAART, or highly active antiretroviral therapy, the famed "triple cocktail" approach to combating the virus. Over time, HAART therapies become so exacting, most cases of HIV rarely progress to AIDS, thereby significantly decreasing the mortality rate.

CYBERSPACE

I don't know if I'm allowed to use the word "cyberspace" anymore. I haven't heard it in a long time, perhaps years. We have no reason to continue to think of the internet as a location, or place to visit, in the way we once did. Now we regard it as a natural resource, as something that simply is, like oxygen or ocean water. And speaking of water: we no longer "surf" it either. "Surf the web" and "World Wide Web" and "weblog" have all gone the way of the dodo and disappeared from the daily vernacular, along with "information superhighway" and "microblogging."

An entry on Wikipedia catalogs old internet metaphors and describes their importance:

Internet metaphors provide users and researchers of the Internet a structure for understanding and communicating its various functions, uses, and experiences. An advantage of employing metaphors is that they permit individuals to visualize an abstract concept or phenomenon with which they have limited experience by comparing it with a concrete, well-understood concept such as physical movement through space. . . . Over time these metaphors have become embedded in cultural communications, subconsciously shaping the cognitive frameworks and perceptions of users who guide the Internet's future development.

INFECTION OF IMAGES

"What do you think Mom will look like now?"

"I don't know."

"Do you remember her?"

"Not really. Only from that little movie we saw."

—*Paris, Texas*

It must have been something when characters in films began to say things like this, when our celluloid creations began to echo what we had privately experienced but had never heard out in the world before. What I mean is: it must have been a vibe when popular culture started acknowledging this new, contemporary condition.

I imagine this misremembering was in circulation long before it was ever projected on the Big Screen, and for reasons unknown to me, I can't help but wonder what it felt like back then to have such an intimate thought reflected at you, before we openly talked about the infection of images.

NIGHTTIME REFRACTION

I leave Netflix on auto-play until the battery dies or the sun comes out. I swim in and out of the sheets, become drowsy during an episode of something only to open my eyes every few hours to find the same characters in completely different scenarios, seasons, jobs, and relationship configurations. The night becomes a montage of unrelated details: a close-up of a hand adjusting a cuff link, a two-shot of a man and a woman toasting pints in a dingy neon-lit bar, a panorama of the Seattle skyline, an over-the-shoulder that racks focus to a woman in the background biting her lip, a patient having a seizure in an MRI machine, a man playing "Georgia" on an upright piano . . . Plots and characters are splintered off from their original episodes and these shards interlock into an irreproducible film dictated by the closing of my eyelids. Snippets of dialogue chirp in the background like forest insects. The activity of the screen glows at my back or into my face, manicured reality blurs with real life, and the mixture infects me. These scripted presences are reliable. They fill the emptiness of my bed. They make me laugh and everything in them means something; life always means more on television. People are not afraid to say what's in their hearts, and if they are, they get over themselves because they've only got forty-four minutes to get to the point. These late-night immersions into fiction are a coping mechanism, albeit a shitty one, but it works for me, for now. When I'm riding the wave between levels of consciousness, I involuntarily absorb the fragments of what I'm watching down into my genomic layer. I latch on to them and the succession of moving pictures is converted into A-T-C-G, a ribbon of letters that seamlessly joins into my own.

For years I've slept in choppy patterns, and I wonder if I will ever feel normal enough to take my eight hours in my stride, like I deserve them. The time now is 3:28 A.M., and I feel my throat start to narrow and constrict. My breathing grows tight. The tide of anxiety is rising and I use my old tactic of going back to the beginning of my symptoms and sleeplessness. Retracing "the narrative" gives me a sense of control and that can sometimes halt the physiological aspects of the panic, so I pull on the rope of memory. My hands curl around the bristly knots and search for the very first one in this particular sequence as stray fibers pierce my skin. I try to locate the moment when this all began, but as usual, I don't get very far.

I check the time again and peel out of the sheets as if removing a wet membrane. In the living room, waiting for the kettle to boil, I stick my fingers between the slats of the blinds to see what sort of moon it is tonight, but it doesn't seem to be there. Instead, I see the corner streetlamp with a little moth fluttering underneath it. A chill twists down into my stomach. I become full of goose bumps and leave the blinds alone. The kettle flicks off and my body flinches in reaction to the sound. I will never understand how the night transforms the ordinary into something eerie. It must have something to do with the shift in our vision. Different receptors in the eye become active in low-light situations and perhaps this change has a subtle effect on cognition and thought. Our perceptions are different because the electrochemical activity inside our body actually is different.

I place two bags of chamomile in a mug and creep back to bed, hunker down with my laptop, and open Netflix. I let an episode of *White Collar* play without the audio, the sparkling images of blue-skied Manhattan perfectly meaningless and strange, like ads in a magazine running into one another.

After a while I split myself in two. The tea works, setting my nervous system in the present, but my mind keeps wandering into that other timeline. It keeps counting the knots . . . I know the way to end this, or so I've been told, is very neat, clinical in fact. All it would take would be a real, true admission of feeling to a friend or "trained professional," but even now, just thinking the words "I miss my mom" sends such a wave of sorrow into my heart I—

Unmute the show and watch a scene where debonair con man Neal Caffrey forges an oil painting in a single afternoon. There's Neal in his undershirt, in his Upper East Side bachelor pad, studying a Degas and imitating the brushstrokes across a blank canvas propped theatrically on an easel. A "passage of time" montage ensues, with the forgery developing more and more with each cut as the sun makes its late afternoon descent. By the time Neal finishes, a raspberry sunset melts across the sky, the pinpricks of stars appearing at the top of the screen.

WHERE IS IT?

Internationally renowned crime fiction author James Ellroy writes that Los Angeles is "epidemically everywhere and discernible only in glimpses."

VIRAL ETYMOLOGY

The Latin definition of "virus" had three clear strains of meaning, as if the word, like the entity, knew its greatest chance of survival was through fracturing across multiple channels. These three strains persist in today's English definition, allowing the virus concept to be deployed across a large berth. Meaning slime, venom, or poison, virus (curiously) describes both malignant and neutral situations.

"Slime" speaks more to the texture of a substance than its effect, so a virus might be semen in one case, or hemlock in another. It is also the liquid dripping off a snake fang, a lethal venom to some, a healing tonic to others. If the etymology gives us any insight into the evolution of our own current viral situations it is only that of freedom. There are many directions a virus could go in, its essence not fixed in limestone like a fossilized sea star, its delicate legs so gently compressed in sediment it looks like the first photograph ever taken.

E FOR EBOLA?

Over Labor Day weekend in 1995, computer programmer Pierre Omidyar launches AuctionWeb as part of his personal website, ebay.com. AuctionWeb facilitates the exchange or sale of goods between consumers, implementing, as its name suggests, a bidding-style purchasing system. It is "dedicated to bringing together buyers and sellers in an honest and open marketplace." As the e-commerce space is mostly undeveloped, interest in AuctionWeb surges, completely overshadowing the other content on Omidyar's website, such as a section devoted to the Ebola virus.

MACULAR DEGENERATION

If you draw a horizontal line from the pupil straight backward into the skull, you will find the macula, or the center of the retina. It is a region of tightly packed photoreceptors that enable "high-acuity vision" or detailed, color vision in daylight. The macula itself has a center called the fovea, which is further subdivided into unique structures. The collection of all the macular aspects forms a tiny island in the geography of the eyeball, but its contribution to the visual capacity of the brain is overwhelming. The macula is thus primarily responsible for our sense of sight. Unfortunately, it isn't sound. It grows vulnerable, particularly in old age, making macular degeneration a common affliction among senior citizens. There are two types:

- In dry age-related macular degeneration, little grains or crystals of cellular debris called drusen form between the retina and the vascular layer of the eye known as the choroid. The accumulation of drusen scars the macula, eventually causing damage to the photoreceptors.

- In wet age-related macular degeneration, there is a spontaneous overgrowth of delicate blood vessels in the choroid. These wisplike vessels tend to break, causing a leakage of blood and proteins that "stain" and damage the retina.

In both instances the patient's central vision is lost while their peripheral remains intact.

After diagnosis, patients are issued Amsler grids to help assess the progression of the disease. Per their name, these diagrams are grids of black lines set on white sheets of paper. If at any point the lines appear wavy or contorted, patients are advised to seek immediate medical attention.

EXPLOSIVE CONTAGION IN NETWORKS

A research paper titled "Explosive Contagion in Networks" was caught in a frenzy of media attention in February 2016. Clickbait articles bearing bombastic headlines like "There's a Formula for How to Break the Internet" declared that the next big viral sensation could be predicted and even manufactured. In actuality, the purpose of the research was simply to demonstrate through mathematics how "synergistic mechanisms," or the online relationships between people, could trigger a viral explosion.

The "going viral" metaphor is briefly touched upon in the opening of the paper:

> Communication between pairs of individuals constitutes the basic building block of macroscopic contagion and dissemination of social phenomena such as behaviors, ideas or products. The mathematical formulation for social diffusion is reminiscent of the spread of infectious diseases and it is indeed common to use the term *viral* to refer to the rapid advent of a product or an idea. Following this analogy, compartmental epidemic models such as the Susceptible-Infected-Susceptible (SIS) or the Susceptible-Infected-Recovered (SIR) are often used to describe the dynamics of the transmission of social phenomena.

From this point on the text becomes dense, burly, and equation based, focusing primarily on the hiccups and fissures within networks that indirectly cause viral tsunamis. It does not provide a formula for breaking the internet, nor does it ever acknowledge how outrageously strange it is to apply epidemiological models to, say, YouTube videos. This, after all, doesn't follow. It is not a logical maneuver to apply mathematical formulations of organic matter to the spread of a Billie Eilish song, and yet: we do. The correspondence even seems to come naturally, like breathing. We never question it. But even more peculiar than this instinct is the fact that *it works*. Epidemic models work in the digital realm, so: was "going viral" ever a metaphor or just an evolutionary term?

DOPPELGÄNGER

"Metaphor: a figure of speech offering one thing for another. A stand-in. A stuntman. A body double."
— *Everything Now: Lessons from*
the City-State of Los Angeles
by ROSECRANS BALDWIN

UNKNOWN ESSENCE

At the library I came across a seventeenth-century definition of "virus" written by a Scandinavian monk. The monk defined the virus as "a principle unknown in its essence, and inaccessible to our senses; but inherent in some animal humors and able to transmit the disease which has produced it."

When I left the library the definition was still attached to me. As I rode home on the bus, I kept revolving it in my mind, and when the trees began to look familiar, marking the return to my neighborhood, the words crushed into a point. "Unknown essence, inaccessible to our senses" defines the virality of the present with a freakish precision. The essence of a trending tweet or a TikTok dance is a complete mystery. We know our reaction to the thing, but not the thing-in-itself. There is no immediate comprehension of, say, why one cat on Instagram trends over another. We recognize a posting format or file type, we understand the casing of an idea, but not its core, which, if it ever existed, surely becomes lost in a series of reposts.

When I alighted at Old Street and walked up Commercial Road there was something else scratching at me about these words. I tried to shake it off, but as I kept walking it sank in further and upset my rhythmic pace. I realized "a principle unknown in its essence" creates a void by way of inversion: my mind cuts open a space for an idea, the principle, only to find there's nothing inside it. As a consequence, I shift my attention to this emptiness, this unknown essence, and, strangely, it becomes visible. It clicks into focus as a quantity of volume, appearing through a feat of reverse engineering.

These thoughts occupied me until I reached the pub on my corner. When I looked in the windows it was full of red faces brimming with cheer, caught up in conversation and desire. I walked on by to my front door and as I pulled it open and started up the stairs all I could think was how extraordinary it is that words could create antimatter, make you see something that was never there in the first place.

COME ON AND SAFARI WITH ME

In 1996 approximately forty-five million people "surf the web."

SOME THINGS ABOUT METAPHOR

1. People will tell you that it's obvious, but it's not. It operates under the surfaces of things and moves them along. You aren't meant to see it, only its currents, only the comparison between X and Y. The actual apparatus is, strictly speaking, invisible.

2. It works by misdirection: while it demonstrates there is nothing up its sleeves, you pay attention to the garment and forget about the arms inside conducting the manipulation, and all metaphor is, in some way or the other, about the body—

3. We tend to perceive the body as a container. We put things into it, and things come out of it, and all of our blood and organs are prevented from sloshing around by a fascial suit. Our epidermis creates a clear boundary between our internal and external environments, and we use this framework to navigate the world. In essence, we imprint our bodily awareness onto space. In their seminal text *Metaphors We Live By*, linguists George Lakoff and Mark Johnson write that even "when things have no distinct boundaries, we often project boundaries upon them—conceptualizing them as entities and often as containers (for example, forests, clearings, clouds, etc.)."

4. To keep it simple: there are no metaphors that exist beyond our plasma, nerves, and bipedal orientation. It all collapses back to a nervous system, and sure, this is obvious, but how many people can honestly say they think of love as a container they fall into (or out of)?

5. The photograph *Leap into the Void* was taken in 1960. It captures the moment artist Yves Klein ejected himself out of a second-story window and into thin air. His dynamic physicality of arched back and sprawled limbs is meant to convey flight and a slagging off of gravity, but the picture itself seems to suggest something more about falling. Also, the whole thing is a lie. The image is a composite of two different negatives: one of the

empty street, and the other of the "leap" where beneath Klein's body a white tarpaulin awaits his fall. Distributed on newspaper broadsheets, the composite image circulated around Paris as breaking news. If ever a situation was emblematic of metaphor it is this one.

6. On "Metaphor in Literature," a webpage, there is a list of quotes by Ralph Waldo Emerson, Friedrich Nietzsche, André Breton, and Robert Frost. Some of the quotes approach metaphor directly while others take an oblique view, describing the situation of metaphor without using its name. For example, in the middle of the list there are a few lines by the Soviet theorist Viktor Shklovsky: "An image is not a permanent referent for those mutable complexities of life which are revealed through it; its purpose is not to make us perceive meaning, but to create a special perception of the object," but a photograph, in a material sense, *is permanent*. It is a physical object that one might say *contains* an image—

7. Postcards are images, often photographs, that travel the world. We hardly use them anymore, but thirty, forty, fifty years ago you could get a sliver of Palm Springs, Palm Beach, and Palm Desert delivered straight to your door. Postcards are pieces of reality chiseled out of one location and sent onward to another, pieces you can hold in your hand or tape to a wall. The neon of the Flamingo Casino, the spray of Niagara Falls, the brittle walls of the Colosseum, all these iconic scenes and places are in transit via their posted images. The images travel, sail, and fly, and the cities they depict are channeled through them like electrical conduits, like the very first motion pictures.

8. Anne Carson writes, "Aristotle says that metaphor causes the mind to experience itself in the act of making a mistake." Metaphors interrupt one's natural flow of thought, causing it to brake, reverse, and continue in new directions. The sensation of the mind experiencing itself, whether or not mistakes are involved, is sublime, like the salt of the Mediterranean suspending your body over its waves.

9. Aristotle writes, "To make good metaphors implies an eye for resemblances," and believes mastery of the form is indicative of brilliance. He ties genius to the optical, the words "eye" and "resemblances" jutting out of the statement to accentuate the point that creating metaphor is reliant on a certain kind of vision: the ability to see the connections between objects with no apparent similarities.

10. To sink under the surfaces of things, to get inside their skeletons and psyches, to find connections, one must sit still and observe.

11. I read a novel about a guy looking back on his childhood from the vantage point of his twilight years. Speaking in the first person, the narrator recounts his friendship with a young boy called Cletus. They meet one afternoon in the construction frame of a house and play around in the undefined space of it. The two become fast friends, in that effortless way only young boys can, and they make a habit of returning to the house day after day to regard its progress. One afternoon, Cletus doesn't show. It transpires that his father has taken his own life after committing a murder, and the narrator never really sees him

again except once, many years later, in the hallway of a gigantic public high school. The two boys look at each other just as the bell rings and: that's it. The narrator lets the glance go, and it's haunted him ever since. His only means of reckoning with this regret is writing. He goes back in time and composes a speculative history of Cletus's life around the time of the homicide. The novel then shifts and dissolves into this imagined history, but in the last few pages the narrator makes a personal admission: he's never gotten over his own mother's death. The whole activity of composing his friend's narrative was nothing but a smoke screen. The narrator was really trying to write about himself. He was trying to tell you about his pain.

12. How you put two pieces of the world together shows how you see something. It discloses a relationship between you and two elements, so if the metaphor for your loss is a long country road, or the wind, or if you talk about an image in terms of virality, you give something of yourself away.

   But: maybe that's obvious?

13. A postcard contains both an image and a message. It puts two elements together to construct an experience.

14. Wish you were here.

ALBUM AMICORUM

The first albums were bibles. During the fifteenth century, the aristocracy of Northern Europe sent their offspring to study at institutions across the continent. The students carried their family bibles with them on these expeditions, and at the end of their studies, tutors and mentors were asked to inscribe messages in blank areas of the pages. Commonly written in Latin or Greek, the messages were both sentimental and practical, often emphasizing the student's achievements. Over time, these bibles began to function as CVs or credentials, as the messages were read as endorsements of the student's character. Later bibles were printed with blank pages specifically for the collection of these notes, which over the years had evolved to include illustrations, poems, locks of hair, and painted coats of arms. The trend culminated in the printing of blank notebooks. The Germans and Dutch popularized their use, calling them "album amicorum," or "album of friends."

The impulse to take your friends with you through time is painfully romantic, and yet, not ridiculous; that every face you've ever loved or shared an affinity with could exist within the space of a single book suggests a desire to keep all of time present around you. What could be more sincere than that? The desire to hold on to everything always?

CLOSEST LIVING RELATIVE

On a first date at a vegan restaurant, he prods me about my parents. It's not first-date material but I kind of gush it all out, and now ol' freelance producer Kevin wants to know what they did for a living, and how old they were when they died, and how they got AIDS. I don't know the answer to any of these questions. I push some wilted rocket leaves around my plate, mix them up with some Soyrizo, take a sip of (biodynamic) wine. The truth is: I have no idea how to tell another person that I feel closer to the thing that killed them than to either of their identities because that thing still exists. It still roams the Earth. It is my closest living relative.

SHARDS

1. The Boss is waiting for him in a lobby decked out in Christmas decorations. The lobby happens to belong to the White House. Garlands of holly and ivy are woven around banisters, and delicate white lights cast a warm glow across the interior. A fire burns in the background. When the Guy shuffles past the Boss, preoccupied with things on his mind, the Boss calls out to him, "How did it go?" The Guy turns around with a touched sort of bafflement across his face. "Did you wait here for me?" The Guy has spent all day in a mandatory counseling session with a traumatologist because he was recently shot in the chest and instead of simply dealing with it, he keeps being a dick to other people. The Boss understands this because he too has been in dark places, dealt with demons, and been forced into professional help. The Guy starts rattling off some smartass remarks about the session, and the Boss lets him go on for a while before whipping off his glasses and meeting him in the center of the room. Then they just stand there looking at each other in silence. After a moment the Boss says:

> This guy's walking down the street when he falls in a hole. The walls are so steep he can't get out. A doctor passes by and the guy shouts up, "Hey you. Can you help me out?" The doctor writes a prescription, throws it down in the hole, and moves on. Then a priest comes

along and the guy shouts up, "Father, I'm down in this hole, can you help me out?" The priest writes out a prayer, throws it down in the hole, and moves on. Then a friend walks by. "Hey, Joe, it's me, can you help me out?" And the friend jumps in the hole. Our guy says, "Are you stupid? Now we're both down here." The friend says, "Yeah, but I've been down here before and I know the way out."

2. A high-powered litigator sits in his office after hours drinking wine out of a red mug. The wine is from an eight-thousand-dollar bottle, a gift from a crush, a young law student whose father happens to be the third-richest man in the world. The Litigator could give a fuck. He is in love with someone else, a married woman with two kids whose husband is in the process of running for public office. In other words, "It's complicated." The Litigator takes a sip of the wine, swishes it in his mouth, and, after a beat, stands up. He straightens his tie, buttons his jacket, and calls the Woman on his cellphone. She picks up and he says, "I was just thinking—I don't want to go through life and think something didn't happen just because I didn't make myself clear." Of course, she can't hear a single thing he's saying. There's too much noise at her husband's press conference to catch the words, so she ducks down a corridor, leans against a doorway, and strains her auditory faculties to grasp what is turning into a declaration of love. But right before his full admission, she shuts him down: "Show me a plan . . . Poetry is easy. It's the parent-teacher conferences that are hard." She hangs up. He paces. Moodily, he prowls into another room and calls her right back. He switches on the television as her voice-

mail picks up and there she is onscreen at the conference, look-ing regal next to her husband. The broadcast makes the Litigator swallow his words. He apologizes for the previous conversation, says he's "dropping it," and hangs up. Marching back to his office, he moves like he has physically slammed shut an entire chapter of his life. His gait is assured, certain, quick, but then he suddenly freezes. He reaches for his phone and calls her for a *third time*. He stares out his window, looking at the glimmering high-rises of Chicago, and says, "No, you know what? I'm not just dropping this. You wanna know my plan? My plan is I love you, okay? I've probably loved you ever since Georgetown. So phone me. I'll meet you anywhere, and we will make a plan."

3. Two surgical interns are across the street from the hospital at a bar called Emerald City. They sit at the counter. One intern, in a Dartmouth sweatshirt, has a series of shot glasses in front of her spread haphazardly among peanut shells. The other intern, in a leather jacket, drinks nothing, but fidgets with her hands. She is accidentally pregnant by her boss, a hotshot cardio-thoracic surgeon. Actually, both interns, despite being set up as healthy rivals with opposing emotional makeups, have been fucking their bosses, and Dartmouth Intern has spent the after-noon in surgery with her boss's/boyfriend's/now most likely ex-boyfriend's Surprise Wife. It has been a long day, hence con-vening at the bar. Leather Jacket Intern starts to explain that she couldn't confirm her abortion appointment without an emergency contact: "Anyway, I put your name down. That's why I told you I'm pregnant. You're my person—"
   "I am?"

"Yeah, you are. Whatever—"

"Whatever," Dartmouth Intern parrots back in the same deadpan, too-cool-for-school intonation as her friend, but a smile breaks across her face.

While eating a peanut, Leather Jacket Intern says, "He dumped me," and Dartmouth Intern just melts into her, lays her head on her shoulder, wraps her arms around her back, and says, "I'm your person."

4. The Captain of a battleship is having a candid conversation with the maintenance engineer of the fighter spacecrafts. The engineer, or the Chief, as he's called, has recently found out that the love of his life is not biologically human but a member of a robot race responsible for the annihilation of 99.999 percent of humanity. Obviously, this brings up a lot of philosophical issues, least of which is: can a man love a machine? The conversation unfolds in the Captain's quarters, a mixture of blinking consoles and antique navigational equipment. The Captain is an older fellow with a lumbering walk and a soft, thoughtful manner of speech. He is currently recovering from a chest wound inflicted by the aforementioned Robot Lover, who shot him three times at close range. He sweats as he maneuvers behind his desk, his dog tags glistening against the skin of his neck. Once settled he gently asks, "Did you love her?" The question pierces the Chief in all the wrong places, and he snaps, letting rage take hold of his senses. But after a moment, his face lets go of the blood boiling beneath it and he considers the question. "I thought I did." The Captain inhales and then gently responds, "Well, when you think you love somebody, you love them. That's what love is. Thoughts."

5. In a car on a desolate highway, two police detectives in their early forties drive underneath a silver sky. The skeletons of trees appear in and out of the windows, their black naked branches reaching out like arthritic arms. One detective, who has the face of an old shoe, works on knotting his tie. He moves his hands in slow motion as if he's never performed the task before, but it is just because his mind is elsewhere, like on the twenty-year-old he's banging alongside his wife of ten years. To further complicate matters, the Shoe-Faced Detective actually rescued the twenty-year-old from a cult when she was a child. Their paths crossed again recently at a cellphone shop in a strip mall. He asks his partner, "Think a man can love two women at once? I mean, be in love with them?"

The other detective, with a sandpaper soul, responds, "I don't think that man can love, at least not in the way that he means. Inadequacies of reality always set in . . ." His eyes stretch through the windshield, surveying the terrain before he absentmindedly remarks, "Place is gonna be underwater in thirty years."

He cracks open a silver Zippo lighter, lights a cigarette, and drags on it in a way that makes you ache for one regardless of your stance on the habit. As smoke curls through the car interior, they go in deep for a few more seconds: "Do you wonder ever if you're a bad man?"

6. At a piano bar in Seattle, three men, all related, sit at the counter staring into their cups. The retired cop father has a beer, the eldest son a martini, and his brother a glass of white wine. A bowl of nuts sits in front of them. Earlier that day, all their girlfriends broke up with them, and now they sit, single, awash

in feelings of hopelessness. In terms of love, they seem to share a genetic predisposition toward failure. A bartender in a black vest and a bow tie polishes glasses as the gentle notes of the piano waft in. The Father suddenly perks up and hobbles on his cane over to the instrument. He requests "Ac-Cent-Tchu-Ate the Positive," but the guy at the keyboard admits he's not the hired musician, just some doofus who sat down to tinker. The Father, visibly crestfallen, asks if there's anything he can play. It transpires that Doofus has a repertoire of three songs: "Happy Birthday," "America the Beautiful," and "Goldfinger." The Father selects "Goldfinger" and calls to his boys to come over and join him. The Brothers groan, look at each other, and then roll their eyes to the heavens. They are *so* above this, but they slump off their stools and stand behind the keyboard as the intro plays. The Dad starts feeding the lyrics to the Brothers in breathy sentences ahead of the music, trying to jog their memories. "You knew the words when you were little!" The Brothers look like they would rather be dead animals on the side of the road than participate in this. "He's the man, the man with the Midas touch," and, "Such a cold finger," and then, just like that, the walls come down. The words come back and the Brothers go with them, fingers pointing, feet stamping as they surrender to the utter absurdity of being over forty and single, and singing a Bond theme tune aloud with their father in a piano bar.

IF YOU'RE WONDERING WHY
THOSE SCENES ARE HERE

These people are my family.

CHRONICLE OF LINKS

On December 17, 1997, the term "weblog" is coined by Jorn Barger, editor and founder of robotwisdom.com. Inspired by recent advents in online publishing tools, Barger begins posting regular, essay-like writings on his site. These posts feature a myriad of hyperlinks that tend to chronicle or "log" Barger's daily journeys throughout the web, hence the terminology WebLog, or weblog. The term is shortened to "blog" in 1999 by Peter Merholz, on his blog peterme.com. In 1999, according to a list compiled by Jesse James Garrett, a future UX designer, there are twenty-three active blogs. By 2006 this number will have increased to fifty million, according to Technorati, a search engine devoted to blogs.

HUNTER OR PREY

Of course, in these Tinder situations, I can never tell if I'm the hunter or the prey. Swiping at men, narrowing the field, selecting a target, firing off a text, is this not the echo of bloodlust? It feels the same as prowling the jungle in search of one's next meal, and isn't it, too, the same crapshoot? Finding love or finding food are two experiences reliant on chance. A hybrid virus spilling over into a human: another experience dictated by chance. If the underlying factor of these situations is actually the same, and if the gestures are the same, maybe I am indeed the hunter. The role replicated in different scenarios creates a thread through time, connecting person to person. But, if this is the case, doesn't this also make me a descendant of the Hunter from 120 years ago? If you wanted, couldn't you draw a line from him to me?

COLLECTIVE HALLUCINATION

"The Internet Protocol suite is a freely available set of standards for how digital devices and the software running upon them might talk to one another, and the internet exists because the makers of those devices and software, and the networks to which they're connected, have decided to implement those standards. The internet is a collective hallucination that functions because millions of people and companies believe in it."

— "Internet" by JONATHAN ZITTRAIN

VIRUSES MANIPULATE BEHAVIOR

A disconcerting feature of certain viruses is their ability to manipulate behavior. The most commonly cited example of this is hydrophobia, which is caused by the rabies virus. The reservoir of the virus is located in the host's salivary glands, so the consumption and consequent swallowing of any liquid severely compromises viral production. To circumvent this issue, the host begins to experience spasms of the larynx and throat, which ultimately inhibits the intake of fluids. This gradually evolves into a fear of water, as the spasms and imbibing become inextricably (and feverishly) linked in the host's mind. Wikipedia explains, "Since the infected individual cannot swallow saliva and water, the virus has a much higher chance of being transmitted, because it multiplies and accumulates in the salivary glands and is transmitted through biting."

The comedy version of behavior modification occurs with the flu virus. A 2010 study showed that people were more up for going out (to bars) in the forty-eight hours following viral exposure than they had been previously. In the postexposure, presymptomatic period, infected subjects exhibited a desire and eagerness to hit the town in a way that was demonstrably different to their pre-infected states; and of course, it is during this window that a person is at their most contagious. The virus has evolved to pluck at our social instincts, strumming them so it too can mingle.

BACK-TO-SCHOOL NIGHT

Mr. Keller was in his early sixties and suffered from macular degeneration, which made him an odd choice for a high school telecommunications teacher. His visual impairment, like Nivia's, was severe, with his central channel of vision all but destroyed by the disease. When the two met at back-to-school night this is primarily what they discussed after the obligatory remarks on my performance as a student:

"She's a good egg, a good student," Keller said.

"Yes. She is a very good girl except sometimes she has these moods." At which point Nivia made her hands into claws, hunched her upper body, and growled in an approximation of a feral cat.

Keller gave a hearty laugh, and I felt all the blood in my body instantly explode through whatever tubes and veins were containing it.

"What part of her is like—" And he reproduced the gesture, at which point, I died. Nivia's motions had somehow been so pronounced that even a person declared blind by the state of California could "see" them and then vividly reproduce them.

"She gets it from her father. He was Irish . . . Her mother, though, was never like that. Always cheerful, always bright . . . she skipped two grades in elementary school."

Nivia was attempting to convey that all my negative traits, or "depressive tendencies," were inherited from my father's side, and thus completely unrelated to her bloodline. My voice wanted to crackle through at that moment to correct her about my blue moods, which were caused by grief and not genetic predisposition, but instead I stood there like a petrified tree until they forgot I was there. I was adept at dissolving my personality to such a degree I could fade out into the background with hardly anyone noticing, and I did this as the conversation trailed into their respective diagnoses.

When we left the computer lab, we walked slowly through the empty hall, moving quietly, like a pair of clouds. For whatever reason, turnout for back-to-school night was dismal that year, and between the emptiness of the event and the teachers seeing me outside of a "normal" parental configuration, a hush grew around us that made everything feel not quite real.

MAKING A NAME

On January 17, 1998, the news aggregation website Drudge Report is the first outlet to break news of the Monica Lewinsky scandal. This is arguably the first story to legitimize web-based journalism.

Later that year, a search engine that yields results from a system based on academic citation is launched. On Google, sites are ranked algorithmically by the quality and quantity of links that trace back to, or "cite," them. Just as the validity of a scientific research paper is strengthened by the number of studies that reference it, Google's search results are rendered more valuable than those of its competitors since they are generated from the architecture of the web itself. While other search engines produce results solely through text and keyword matches, Google analyzes the link structure of the web to derive relevancy for its hits.

EXOSKELETONS

All I can say is the sensation of having witnessed the life cycles of a metaphor is heavy. It makes me feel age, or the actual physical weight of the years that have passed from when an idea was new to now, and if I pause and look around, I see the exoskeletons of terms piling up around me in some desert of time I always heard people talk about but didn't realize I, too, was wandering in.

CAT VIDEOS

An artificial brain composed of sixteen thousand computer cores taught itself, after viewing ten million YouTube clips, what a cat is. The brain, or neural network, was constructed in 2011 at Google's mysterious X lab, and was unleashed on YouTube in 2012 for a brief seventy-two-hour period. During this time it was free to explore video content without limitation. Meaning, the network had not been instructed to do or find anything in particular, but could browse just as a person might, and somehow, through this browsing, "it basically invented the concept of a cat," as Google fellow Jeff Dean told *The New York Times*. Previously, the network was a tabula rasa consisting only of a "deep learning" algorithm. After exposure to content, the network forged a vocabulary from the most commonly featured objects in videos. In essence, it was able to teach itself, through the consumption of vast amounts of unlabeled data, to recognize commonalities and categorize them appropriately. At the conclusion of the experiment, the network could reliably identify cats in images even if those images were distorted or pixelated. The greater application of this technology is naturally facial recognition software. The takeaway outlined in the research paper states, "Our experimental results reveal that it is possible to train a face detector without having to label images as containing a face or not." The network is purportedly composed of one billion connections.

All of this is a marvel, yet aspects of it remain unsettling. First, should content on the web, particularly that of YouTube, be a training model for a synthetic brain? Doesn't this just solidify the wonkiness and surreality of online content into something . . . legitimate? And second: cats. Aside from being brilliant PR, isn't this a tad eerie? Why should a fledgling intelligence so accurately parallel our own desires? Of course, it is learning through us and what we create, but how did it truly identify "cat" before "dog," "chair," or "human"? It is disquieting that the network so effortlessly tapped into one of our core fetishes.

METAPHORS INFLUENCING REASON

If metaphors influence our reasoning in regard to social issues, then by extension, they must influence our reasoning capacity as a whole. Assuming this is the case, then assigning a precise and accurate metaphor to a situation is absolutely critical, for as the Stanford study determined, once a person has been exposed to a particular metaphorical framework they will continue to implement it as a conceptual foundation for further formulations. Information effectively will be siphoned in such a way as to harmonize with the original metaphor, but this has the potential to lead to a contortion of facts. It could cause mental processing to flow away from reality and toward the maintenance of a certain conception. Metaphors therefore must be phenomenally reflective of their targets, and yet . . . they run along the vein. Metaphor is completely reliant on the intersection of life and knowledge. In other words, it is determined by experience.

GRIEF IS A VIRUS

We can say grief is a virus. It penetrates the bloodstream. It sinks into the myelin sheaths of neurons, the calcium of teeth. Temperature becomes deregulated, dampening perceptions, twisting them, folding them, until all sensory info is diluted, as if received from afar. The body aches, barely wants to move. Skin turns clammy and circadian rhythms contort, responding to an unknown baseline. Experience breaks down into a million unrelated particles. The virus chews through the part of the brain that understands time. The linear world becomes a thing of the past.

But to call grief a virus is too easy. To call it anything other than what it *is* too easy. Grief has no metaphor. To give it one or a hundred does nothing but compromise it, or transmute it into a lesser form. Viewing grief through the lens of something else is a way of actually not seeing it, of rendering aspects of it invisible, which is to say: you are cheating.

EXCEPT

Except death sits outside of experience. It cannot be comprehended with the materials of reality. The only way to broach it is in fact through other things, through a transference of energy that occurs between thought and speech:

Words are how we know something happened. We say what we saw and the experience appears.

It becomes observable.

A FEW OBSERVATIONS

1. Inkjet toner, unreturned phone calls, plastic water bottles, wool blazers, his-and-hers sinks, morning commutes, IKEA floor lamps, Ryanair flights, Jesus, box pasta, howling wind, the Royal Oak pub, tap shoes, satellites, Hare Krishnas, insomnia, smallpox, whooping cough, chlamydia, cave paintings, significant others, online dating, hieroglyphics, vegan hair dye, flounders, photo albums, fantasies, dried bubble gum stuck underneath café tables, wordplay, warfare, Louboutin heels, newspapers, Polaroid cameras, cobwebs, Vodafone, shrimp scampi, morons, parquet flooring, dodgeball, lint, peanut M&M's, pickleball, silent film, satellites, stingrays, NFTs, Yule logs, watermelon, wax, vagina-scented candles, Stonehenge, panettone, cinnamon sticks, currywurst, gossip rags, mince pies, dander, hyperpigmentation, mountains, mitochondria, 404 errors, the telegraph, baby teeth, evening skies, painkillers, gin, GeoCities, pride, the Colosseum, drag queens, axe throwing, fax machines, electron microscopes—all came out of the explosion that happened 13.8 billion years ago that also created space and time.

2. Self is the intersection of time, space, and events. It is the circuitry of information running through you, the crisscross of it,

and the gleaming electrical current that keeps it all in motion, that keeps you alive.

3. A book—or an album—is a network of thought, pinching together events and impressions to form a narrative or a lattice of time.

4. The observable universe is a spherical volume centered on the observer. Every location in the universe has its own observable universe.

5. "Language is a virus from outer space."
   —William S. Burroughs

PEER-TO-PEER

Napster, a free peer-to-peer file-sharing service specializing in audio content, launches in the summer of 1999. The platform allows users to exchange music in the form of MP3s, and is comparable to a bazaar in terms of content: everything from the latest album drops to long-lost demos are available. At the height of its power, eighty million users will be active on its network, which will simultaneously devastate the music industry and pave the way for the streaming services of the future.

THE BOOK I WAS WRITING WHEN NIVIA DIED

The book I was writing when Nivia died was about viruses and the spread of ideas. It was about the metaphor "going viral," and our strange need to appeal to a biochemical entity to explain the popularity of memes. Virality seemed to have crept into the vernacular overnight, moving through our mouths and systems during the early aughts, as so many cultural critics have noted, like a pandemic.

I made handwritten timelines of the history of the internet and the history of AIDS and collaged them together to find their moments of intersection in the public consciousness. The timeline grew, became a spine, and vectors of different subjects ranging from microscopy to cat videos extended out from it. These vectors would be contained in the book, and the book itself would be organized in two parts, with the first concentrated on the history of biological viruses, and the second on the viral metaphor. The timeline would rest at the center of the text, showing how the two aspects were inextricably intertwined. I wanted to make a book as if it were a strand of DNA.

The tone would be edgy. Ideas would be "unpacked." Arguments would be deployed with a sexy sleight of hand. Formal tropes of the critical essay would be disrupted by casual yet poetic remarks. The book would fit the style that had been on trend for a while because: the internet.

The deeper I plunged into this material, the more feverish I became. Blood rose to the surface of my skin and thrummed. Dreams, when I had them, were of my computer screen. The project far exceeded my capacities as a scholar and writer. I lacked the discipline to investigate the ideas to their most brutal end points, and yet, I couldn't stop working. The virus was lodged in my skull. I saw it entangled in everything, ceaselessly replicating. I was bearing witness to a vast never-ending network of infection, and then one day it crystalized: the virus is a condition of being human, and its ascension to the cyber realm is simply the realization of its fullest evolutionary potential. We've moved online, the viruses have followed.

Except my book wasn't about this. It also wasn't about viruses or "going viral." It wasn't about the internet. It was not about AIDS. It was not about a literal illness bleeding into the architecture of thought. It was not about a cultural moment. It was not about vision, networks, or observation. It wasn't about metaphor. When I lifted my head from the page, I saw something else—

My book is about grief.

TELEPRESENCE 2

One could argue watching a film or TV show is also a nonphysical experience, akin to "reading" the internet, except we know how to discuss these forms of visual engagement: I tell you a story. I give you a synopsis of what I've seen, and you, as a human, inflate the drama through empathy. You place yourself within the narrative to feel its effects on an intimate level. But what happens online, for whatever reason, doesn't move through us in the same way. Sure, emotion is there, but the communications about the how and the why of it all are completely different. Maybe because information is not art, but an uninterrupted stream with no beginning or end, and thus no location in time.

JESSICA JONES

I wake up from a dream where I'm running away from something. I swipe my arm out from the duvet and jerk my head back into the pillow. A web of sweat covers my face. My heart darts in and around my rib cage like a goldfish. I am throbbing. The phone says 4 A.M. I have been asleep for less than an hour. I flick on the overhead and try to understand that I am in the world, and then I shiver: I check WhatsApp, email, voicemail, Facebook Messenger, and iMessage to make sure Nivia hasn't died, and then I remember that I've done all this before and that she is, in fact, dead.

On my way to the kitchen, I turn on every light in the flat. I pour water into the kettle, press the button, and sit on the sofa while it does its job. I breathe "in a square"—in for four, hold for four, out for four, hold for four—then give up and peek through the blinds to make sure the street hasn't disappeared. It is still there, but unnaturally steady. It doesn't even seem like a strong wind could crack the glass of its surface, and even though nothing is happening my gaze feels intrusive, like it's disturbing the street's own nocturnal reverie. The streetlamp on the corner shines a sodium cone straight into an overflowing bin. A loose newspaper looks like an animal carcass, its pages wet and lumped together, refusing to rustle. Then some lads tumble out of the twenty-four-hour bagel shop on the corner with greasy paper bags crumpled in their fists, and the scene unglues.

The kettle clicks off, and something clicks in my brain. I leave the outside alone, make my tea, and get on with it. Back in bed I reach for my long-term lover, opening Netflix and falling into a series of automatic movements. I browse without taking notice, brush the trackpad like I'm trying to get a stray hair off my fingers, and after a while a thought appears. A memory of a show called *Jessica Jones*.

The credit sequence is an origami of violet shadows that bend and crease into an ink rendition of New York City. A somewhat jazzy electronica tune accompanies the images, and then there is Jones, who seems like your standard jaded P.I., chasing a philander-

ing husband, except she can deadlift a car. She is a P.I. and a super-
hero, though neither the super nor the hero part comes naturally to
her. She tries to keep her power—Herculean strength—on the DL,
which consistently backfires. Things always seem to break in her
presence: jaws, windows, barstools, phones, relationships . . . Her
apartment doubles as her office and fits all the tropes of the detective workplace, from bottles of whiskey stashed in desk drawers to
neglected plants. The pebbled glass window of her front door has
ALIAS INVESTIGATIONS painted across it in gold leaf, but it gets busted
in within the first two minutes of the pilot.

Jones is a raw human who throws one-liners as effectively as
punches. Cynical, brash, the police don't like her. People don't like
her. She does not like herself. Turns out she's an orphan. Her parents and brother died in a car crash she holds herself responsible
for, and suffering from grief, PTSD, and survivor's guilt, she spends
a lot of time in bars being nobody's hero or, rather, fool. Even so,
her heart is in the right place—in pieces, but in a geographically accurate position.

I'm mesmerized. Bands of light emanating from my MacBook
Pro swirl around my eye sockets, and twist down my optic nerve.
Jones breathes like Marlowe. She walks around with the same
swagger and world-weariness, but she's not some lame spin-off or
girl "adaptation" of the role. She is a genetic relation who desper-
ately wants to uphold a moral ideal that is out of step with time.
These two characters lurk on the periphery of society, watching it,
observing it, and then slip through its topographical layers searching for truth. Like Marlowe, Jones wants to operate within the
bounds of the law, but keeps getting pulled into the grime, or as
Marlowe says, "However hard I try to be nice I always end up with
my nose in the dirt and my thumb feeling for somebody's eye."

The greater story arc involves Jones apprehending the supervillain Kilgrave. This task is complicated by the fact that Kilgrave previously abducted her and, through mind control, coerced her to be his sex slave. This history is revealed through a series of flashbacks, which demonstrate Kilgrave's ability to compel anyone to do absolutely anything by uttering a few simple words. Jones was able to escape his clutches during an action-fueled sequence that theoretically killed him . . . except he didn't die, and now he's back to win Jones's hand. He wants a "real relationship" with her, and his method of wooing involves strategically killing as many people as possible to get her attention, or: creating mysteries for her to solve. It is an impossible situation, even without the emotional dimension. Facing a foe whose modus operandi is mind control means there is never any evidence of a crime. It all gets erased. Jones's only recourse is to harvest her own tortured past for clues that might help her unhinge him. This is the genius of the show: the protagonist's power is actually her trauma and she has to face it and transform it in order to save the day.

But on a narrative level, how does mind control work? Unlike other superpowers that exist in the Marvel Universe, of which Jones is a part, mind control lacks a plausible explanation. The origins of superpowers typically fall into one of four categories: alien technology, exposure to radioactive elements, training in mystical arts, or genetic mutation. Mind control doesn't fit comfortably within any of these classifications, but more so there's the issue of how the phenomenon functions: light-speed hypnosis? Sound wave manipulation that disrupts brain activity?

Hypnotized, I keep watching, hoping the origin of Kilgrave's power will be revealed. It happens ten episodes later when his parents show up. Both scientists, and both responsible for his ungodly power through an experiment gone awry (oops), they explain Kilgrave "emits a virus." He literally infects minds around him.

My eyelids start to feel heavy, though part of me is zinging with excitement. Of course it's a bloody virus! A yawn escapes and I let my eyes close. Could anything be more emblematic of our times than this ultimate depiction of "going viral," of power administered through airborne contagion? I try to laugh, but instead I just fall asleep.

ECLIPSE PERIOD

1. There is a period of time when a virus has emptied its genetic contents into a cell but the virus is not, strictly speaking, "there." This moment when the virus is present but also not present is called the eclipse period. In essence, the cell is preparing to manufacture the viral information, but has not yet begun to produce it. If tested for a disease during the eclipse period the results will come back negative even if the patient is infected, making the whole thing a surprisingly existential situation for science. The word "eclipse" is taken from the ancient Greek "ekleipein," meaning "to fail to appear" or "to leave out." The root word implies absence, or a vacancy, which is a strange way for a virus to make an entrance considering it is ultimately an inheritance—not only of an interaction or transaction, but also of eons of information; its code is a tangible record of its history.

2. A person can be left with an inheritance of emotion, but the circumstances that caused it will, after a period, fail to appear.

Once this happens there's no concrete relationship between the input and the output, the past and the present, just traces of feeling that are there but also are not there, since with no points of reference, the meaning dissolves.

BRAVE NEW WORLD

At the turn of the millennium, the World Health Organization estimates 21.8 million people have died of AIDS worldwide. President Clinton, in turn, declares HIV/AIDS a threat to national security.

FERDINAND

On a flight from Calgary to London I watch the horror film *A Quiet Place*. An hour in I've had thrills, starts, scares, and gasps, but now: I'm over it. My attention wanders and falls on the screen of the passenger on my left, a woman in her early seventies. She is watching the animated film *Ferdinand,* about the bull who prefers flowers to fighting. I turn back to Emily Blunt using sign language to convey something of vital importance to her deaf daughter, but again, I can't get involved. My eyes drift around the plane and eventually return to my neighbor's screen. I watch the large, computer-animated bull twirl and frolic in a hyper-green meadow, and I start to cry, only the woman next to me thinks I'm crying because *A Quiet Place* is just so utterly terrifying that she then starts unabashedly staring at my screen. Really, I'm crying over *Ferdinand*. Nivia kept a plastic figurine of a brown cow with the name Ferdinand scribbled in black ink on its torso. It had been a childhood toy of

Vivian's. Improbably, the figurine survived multiple moves and multiple deaths, and I still have it somewhere, in a box.

Silently crying and watching the film, I keep having thoughts like: *My mother loved this story of a gentle creature. My mother was a person in the world who had opinions and preferences. My mother had feelings. My mother was a person—*

These are all such stupid sentences, but they're all I've got.

VIRAL NEUTRAL LANGUAGE

When discussing the actions of viruses, it is nearly impossible not to employ personification. The words "invade," "behave," "voracity," "protest," and "obsession" all inject life force into the virus. Short of equations, we have no neutral language to talk about what viruses do.

In the Venn diagram of living and nonliving characteristics, viruses inhabit the slim middle section, exhibiting attributes of both biological organisms and nonliving substances. For instance, while they possess DNA or RNA like living beings, they are completely unable to metabolize, putting them in the same category as rocks. This inability to generate energy could be read as the motive that drives their infectious behavior except, being inert, they cannot actively strive for or pursue any course of action—even that of survival. Virus particles, virions, drift in the atmosphere, completely innocuous, unless they happen upon the exact set of circumstances that "activate" them, which means their survival is 100 percent dictated by chance. In the event the virion does land on a suitable host, it will immediately "spring to life" and behave with such voracity it seems to consciously uphold the biological imperative. Its obsessive reproduction could be interpreted as a protest against extinction or, nonexistence.

SHOW, DON'T TELL

If you asked me to show you what it was like to grow up under a person like Nivia, I could try to elicit one clear scene exemplary of our complicated dynamic and cut it into a diamond, but I'm not sure how well I would succeed. Here the hackneyed advice given to every writer since the dawn of time resounds in my ear: "Show, don't tell." But relationships, at least for me, don't exist in syntax and punctuation. The mechanics between people lie in another realm altogether, somewhere between instinct, intuition, and knowledge. Better perhaps to say relationships exist on their own frequencies, audible only to the parties involved, and how to describe the frequency of a situation? Isn't it just a wavy line on a page?

POINT OF ORIGIN

If your point of origin is erased, does your life trajectory also vanish?

FIVE SNAPSHOTS OF A TOWN

1. On the edge of town where Walnut dead-ends into Imperial Highway there is a lookout point on top of a hill. People sit here at all times of day and watch jetliners pitch their sleek

bodies into the sky. Concrete benches and tables are fused into the sidewalk and during lunchtime the presence of crustless sandwiches and Tupperware is as common as the contrails over LAX. In the morning, dogs on leashes pull their owners to this stretch and sniff clusters of ice plants cracking through the municipal landscaping. After school, kids run around playing tag, freezing into weird shapes at the sound of takeoff. In the early evenings, the dogs return, and when the sun sinks low, partners stand here holding hands, their chins lifted, scanning for stars. Interspersed between these onlookers are the photographers, professional and amateur alike, who perch their telephoto-lensed cameras on tripods. If you go into any one-hour passport photo shop in the area you will see the photos taken from this vantage point framed on the wall, pictures of Delta and Qantas planes so technically perfect, in air so blue, they look like toy models.

2. There used to be a pharmacy on Main Street with an Rx sign above its entrance like a blue full moon. The automatic doors swung in and out in slow motion, wafting the synthetic aromas of potpourri spice and lavender out into the street. China dolls, jewelry boxes, and glass figurines were all displayed on mirrored shelves that never seemed to acquire dust. The reflections of these objects were further multiplied by mirrors on the wall, creating a silver universe of merchandise. Down in the aisles, rows of pantyhose, nail polishes, and lipsticks were mixed between greeting cards, magazines, and the occasional teddy bear or two dressed in a cap and gown. Prescriptions were serviced in the back where rotating wire racks held paperback mystery thrillers and diet-craze books. The lighting was

brightest there. New fixtures hung and hissed above the white-coat pharmacists, and the glass back-door entrance caught the late afternoon sun as it slid down into the Pacific, those merciless golden rays traveling through the corridor, blinding customers in fold-up chairs waiting for their pills.

3. On Fridays, Saturdays, and Sundays, an organist plays an antique Mighty Wurlitzer from the twenties. Housed in a deep velvet auditorium with an occupancy of 188 seats, the organist cranks out scores to accompany silent film classics. During the overture for each screening, the keyboard of the instrument holds center stage, dominating the space like a control panel for a Soviet missile launch. It runs on a ten-horsepower turbine engine and has over two thousand pipes sprouting out of it like a coral reef organism.

   The nostalgia vibe is in full command here. Two large and intricate crystal chandeliers drip down from the ceiling, and a gold leaf motif cascades down the proscenium like a garland. At any moment a troupe of vaudeville clowns with seltzer bottles might appear, and, in fact, the Old Town Music Hall does book novelty acts. One of them is called Songs of Comfort from Days of Yore, billed as "an afternoon of pot roast for the ears . . ."

4. The public library is situated in a park. Its large windows act as soft membranes, allowing the leafy essence of the surroundings to seep into the bookstacks along with the daylight. Walking inside, you're directed by the flow of the space around the archipelago of the new-release shelves to the main hub of the information desk, where perky librarians assist patrons with

their queries. Behind it are the aisles of reference materials that lead to desks for study. Around the bend is the archive room, which, for some unknown reason, exudes a different aura; the brass handle of the door seems likely to burn your hand if you reach for it. On its dark teal walls are photos of El Segundo in its early days as a settlement for the oil refinery. The pictures are black-and-white, mostly of men covered in dust. A glass display case in the center of the room holds urban planning diagrams on delicate paper yellowing at the edges. The atmosphere is heavy with unsynthesized stories.

5. The mural features two butterflies. One is suspended in flight, and the other is perched on a buckwheat flower. The mural has a definite homemade quality but what makes it unusual are the shadows of the insects. Most objects in murals are completely decontextualized and flattened. Here the shadows release dimensions that are typically folded up or ignored, and their color of not quite gray, not quite charcoal, but a thin blue suggests the creatures' wings are little more than a filter of light.

The butterfly hovers myth-like over the city; that a tiny insect with a wingspan the size of a paper clip should come to symbolize a town tied to the spirit of aviation, with large stakes in the aerospace industry, is a rare convergence of circumstances, but it also reflects a particular folksy interpretation of time and space that did not originate at the Pacific Ocean, but came from elsewhere, across the plains. In all the world, this species of butterfly only exists here.

I am unable to recall a single vivid experience growing up

alongside these things. The environments appear, but only as isolated images: the archway of trees enveloping Arena Street, the industrial carpet of Main Street Video fraying at the counter, the blond hair of the clerk behind it, tinged green from chlorine. I see the art deco façade of the public swimming pool with its huge male and female swimmer duo in concrete relief bordering the entryway, the lights of the baseball field glowing at night. I see bare feet stepping over an ant trail, ceiling fans, dented garage doors, patterns of misfired sprinkler droplets on sidewalks, and bicycles laid out on a front lawn, rusting, but I can't seem to go beyond the scenery into the details of experience.

If I hold myself quiet for long enough, I can sometimes catch a brief sensation, that of walking uphill in afternoon heat. I feel gravity resist me and the weight of several textbooks clunking against my back. Sweat threads my upper arms, and sun pierces the concrete with painfully distinct shadows. Across the street, through the diamonds of a chain-link fence, I watch the high school track team dart around in name-brand athletic wear. I can feel their futures all laid out neatly in front of them, and their mothers in minivans waiting for them in the parking lot.

SOME LITTLE BUG IS GONNA GET YOU SOMEDAY

The ILOVEYOU or Love Bug virus, sent in the form of an email attachment, targets a design flaw in Windows operating systems, ultimately infecting more than forty-five million computers worldwide. The attachment called LOVE-LETTER-FOR-YOU.txt.vbs appears as a lowly text file on account of a setting that obscures the cryptic .vbs extension. Once opened, the virus enthusiastically corrupts files, but to add insult to injury, it also replicates, sending itself to all the contacts listed in the user's address book. The estimated monetary damage of ILOVEYOU is upward of five billion dollars. Interestingly, the genius of the virus comes less from its simple exploitation of an operating system, and more from its ability to prey on human longing; in other words, the success of the virus is dictated by desire and curiosity.

ELECTRON MICROGRAPHS

I google image search "first electron micrographs of viruses" and my screen brims with thumbnails of monochromatic abstractions. The shapes in them are charcoal-like apparitions, shadows and smears that loosely resemble familiar objects: a shoelace curled around itself (Ebola), a cluster of miniature igloos (polio), and a prehistoric approximation of a snowflake (hep C). The background of each micrograph exhibits a strange smoothness, like the powder of the lunar surface, and as I scroll farther down the page my mind inflates with a swarm of associations, trying to grasp what I am looking at, but beyond "broken lengths of fettuccine," I've got nothing.

INTERNET LANGUAGE

How Mr. Keller came to teach at my high school, or what he did before lecturing on "internet language and communication," unfortunately never came up, but he was quite open about other aspects of his life. For instance, my classmates and I knew he was married to a much younger, beautiful blonde, and that they had two perfect-looking, beautiful, blond daughters. He showed us a photograph of them once and the girls were nearly identical in white dresses and pigtail French braids. We also knew that after he was diagnosed with macular degeneration, Keller "retired" from his career and uprooted his family (a different unit from the one just described) to England, where he apprenticed under a bricklayer for a year. In the face of vision loss, he wanted to put some type of technical knowledge into his hands, and after reading an article on the death of bricklaying craftsmanship in the UK, the choice seemed obvious, at least to him.

We never learned if technology entered the picture before or after the bricklaying, but it was clear that it offered Keller a second life. By manipulating the size of graphics and text on computer screens he could maintain a connection to the visual world, which led to his teaching us HTML and other tools of telecommunications in a Cal State LA computer lab. By the end of term each of us had designed personal websites, which ran off the university's servers.

One class period was dedicated to online research. As the lecture began, the classroom lights were switched off, and a slide dimly projected on the pull-down screen came into focus: "How to Use a Search Engine." As the computer terminals hummed, Keller gently guided us through the interfaces of AltaVista and Ask Jeeves on his overhead projector. He went into the minutiae of using quotation marks and "OR" to refine search results into an accurate list of links. Having wrapped up his points quicker than expected, he instructed us, in the last three minutes of class, "Go wild!" He then quickly added that we should search our own full names. "You probably won't get any hits unless you have a state or national sports ranking or were on TV but give it a try!"

And less than a minute later, my father was on screen in a black-and-white photo attached to his *Los Angeles Times* obituary. The headline read, "David McCalden; Failed to Disprove the Holocaust." I scrolled down the page: "McCalden, who also used the name Lewis Brandon, was best known as the director and a founder of the Institute of Historical Review, begun in Torrance in 1978. Among other things, the organization claimed that the Nazi massacre of six million Jews during World War II was a lie." I kept scrolling, and kept typing, and then I found him mentioned on blogs written by "revisionists," neo-Nazis, conservative politicians, and morons, and then all of a sudden class was over and everyone was gone except for me.

When Keller flicked the lights back on, I was trembling. I was not cold, but I was shaking, which posed a problem for exiting the room, so I called out from my desk and asked if I might print a result I had found.

"Maybe," he said. "What is it?"

"A webpage has a little blurb about my dad . . . he died . . ."

"Yes, of course! How could I forget your grandmother's impression! Irish fellow, right?" And he chuckled softly to himself, adjusting his Coke-bottle glasses in the process.

In the reverse of what I experienced on back-to-school night, all the blood in my body drained backward, away from the surface of my skin, and was vacuumed away so violently it was sucked directly into the linoleum of the ground, and through the metal structure of the building's foundation, into the dirt and fault lines of Los Angeles, where it quaked away on the San Andreas, but I managed to crack a smile and nod and get on with the veneer of life to collect the printed obituary. At home I showed it to Nivia, who could only look at it on a device that resembled a microfiche reader; it worked by magnifying text and displaying the results through a live feed on a television screen. When she finished reading, all she could say was, "I'm sorry, darling. At least it is in the past now."

But it wasn't in the past. All the information was right there, right *now*, simmering as if it were alive. And then I understood that the past, the way Nivia had experienced it, was gone from the Earth. Our past would be here forever, mutating in galvanic spheres, always on the other side of the glass, waiting for us.

ESCAPE HYPOTHESIS

Of the three theories of viral evolution, the "escape theory" has remained a splinter in my mind. It has an edge to it: a loose genetic fragment floating in a chemical sea develops a mechanism by which it can once again become whole. Through infection the fragment forms a relationship with an organism, and is no longer a shard of something that was, but a part of something that *is*.

COLLECTIVELY EDITED AND MAINTAINED

Wikipedia, an "online free-content encyclopedia," is launched at the beginning of the aughts. It is a compendium of knowledge that is collectively edited and maintained by volunteers via use of wiki technology, or open-source software that facilitates collaborative creation of webpages. Originally developed as an entertaining counterpart to Nupedia, a slow-growing, *extensively* peer-reviewed online encyclopedia, Wikipedia quickly overshadows it, eventually becoming one of the most cited sources of all time.

METAPHOR DEFINITION

"Metaphor systematically disorganizes the common
sense of things—jumbling together the abstract
with the concrete, the physical with the psychological, the like with the unlike—and reorganizes it into
uncommon combinations."

> —*I Is an Other: The Secret Life of*
> *Metaphor and How It Shapes*
> *the Way We See the World*
> by JAMES GEARY

AMENDMENT

If you replace the word "metaphor" in the sentence above with
"grief," "death," or "loss," the meaning stays exactly the same.

ALL ROADS LEAD TO MY FATHER

He says, "All roads lead to my father," as if it were a song, and the
timbre of his voice suggests he's somehow forgotten that I, too, lost
mine early on. The sentence comes out like a lyric and hangs there
like I might not understand how the waves of one's life could be
traced back to an entire mountain face falling into it but: okay. Loss
is unique to each individual and yet, aside from being born and
breathing, it is the most ubiquitous experience of all. In truth, I am
only irritated that the words did not work their way out of my own
mouth; the roads of my life cannot be reduced to anything as solid
as a person, while my friend, Sam, aches for a particular Man. His
mind. His manner. The way his body filled out a houndstooth

blazer and how, being an engineer, everything he did, including his deployment of language, was soundly constructed. Sam can re-wind everything back to how this person cooked steaks on the grill by the pool no one used, laughed, and drove a car. I have no sense of any of that. It is the feeling of *having* no sense, of a vacancy. Of possessing an iron chamber filled only with air.

The most intriguing thing about my father was his absence. There were perhaps other genuinely interesting elements of his character, but none of them touched me. They didn't even sand down the surface of my skin, whereas his death—not the man, but his passing—chiseled into me, molded me, punctured me, shaped me into something like a person, and to have emptiness bore into you, to have Nothing cause you to grow in a certain way, isn't that like a breakdown of the laws of physics? A paradox in a sci-fi film where the cosmos shrinks down to a pinhead, crumbling all of space and time? So, while Sam talks about his father, I talk about roads and boulevards and where they have taken me. Journeys, faces, bits of facts, viruses, television, towns, microscopes, and art. I talk about images and how they float around in the world like particles.

TRUTH

Hiring a private investigator is harder than you think—

SEEING IS BELIEVING

Seeing is believing. Seeing is believing. Seeing is believing. I keep repeating the phrase as if I could get it to mean something through accumulation. The words however are so empty I can't get them to do anything so, 4:30 A.M. Google—

I scroll hits for sites listing popular idioms, and ones for charities for the visually impaired who use the three words as a marketing slogan. Pages unfurl into religious blog posts on fish, and Abraham wandering through the desert: "Without knowing exactly what he would find as he followed the inspiration of God, Abraham left his home of origin and journeyed through a foreign land. Abraham did not see, yet he believed." Then there's Jesus, burning bushes, and faith: "If faith is not based on what is seen, then on what is it based?" A good question, one I think would go better with a beer, so I grab one out of the fridge, and keep searching until I hit the jackpot on Reddit. A thread explains that "seeing is believing" is actually part of a longer sentence penned by seventeenth-century English church-man Thomas Fuller, who wrote, "Seeing is believing, but feeling is truth." The rest of the thread attempts to decode what Fuller may have meant by the word "feeling." The initial comments are civil, but clearly this is going to go awry at some point. On November 17, 2016, at 10:10 P.M., Felinomancy wrote, "I think people here might confuse 'feeling' (experiencing) with 'feelings' (emotions)," but of course, an emotion *is* an experience and an experience unfolds as feeling—which technically may or may not constitute an emotion. Shrug emoji.

For clarification, I look up Merriam-Webster's definition of emotion:

a conscious mental reaction (such as anger or fear) subjectively experienced as strong feeling usually directed toward a specific object and typically accompanied by physiological and behavioral changes in the body.

If emotion induces physiological change, then the experience of an emotion becomes a concrete reality for the body. In other words:

once embedded in biochemistry, an emotion becomes The Truth, but only an individual one. Beyond this solo configuration there is no way to scientifically determine its existence for anyone else.

The etymology of "emotion" goes back to the 1570s, when it was plucked from the French word "émouvoir," meaning to "excite," "agitate," or "stir up." These terms contextualize emotion as a disturbance, an unsettling force that rustles one's sense of normal. Fear, rage, joy, and happiness all jolt the nervous system out of its daily stupor and trigger self-awareness; the emotions cause a recognition of the pre-disturbed, "neutral" state of being, something so familiar we fail to perceive it on its own. We require the interference of exuberance or sadness to view our own baseline. An emotion, in other words, creates the opportunity for perception.

Delving further down the rabbit hole, I search "perception" on Wikipedia. It is "the organization, identification, and interpretation of sensory information." On the most elementary level this involves the transformation of a stimulus into neuronal activity. On psychological, philosophical, and cognitive levels, the processing of that neuronal activity is then affected by "a person's concepts and expectations (or knowledge)," and "restorative and selective mechanisms (such as attention)," which means there is currently no way to determine how one's belief system or concentration might influence the perception of the color red, or of Haydn's Keyboard Concerto no. 11 in D Major. We don't know much about this, or even if our perception of a stimulus is correct. There is no way to confirm the correlation between a perceived stimulus and its actual form because our understanding of "objective reality" is based on perception. Mental "processes produce the experiential phenomena but they are not the phenomena," so whatever we are sensing or feeling is probably just our mind.

An issue of *Scientific American* devoted to illusions begins, "We are wired to analyze the constant flood of information from our senses and organize that input into a rational interpretation of our world." A rational interpretation is necessarily a narrative interpretation bound to the logic of causality. Storytelling thus begins on the cellular level. It's in our blood. We can't help it.

AUTONOMOUS PROTECTION

In 2003, the International Partnership for Microbicides receives a sixty-million-dollar grant from the Bill and Melinda Gates Foundation to continue researching the prevention of HIV through microbicides, or organic compounds. The IPM is a nonprofit organization whose mission is "to provide women with safe, effective and affordable products they can use to protect themselves against HIV infection." According to the WHO, "Unlike male or female condoms, microbicides are a potential preventive option that women can easily control and do not require the cooperation, consent, or even knowledge of the partner."

SELF-PRESERVATION INSTINCT

I wake up with my stomach on fire. It is the kind of pain where even the mere thought of touching the affected area causes you to recoil. The impulse to self-soothe in the fetal position must be fought. The distress of finding my dad online has shaken me, literally, to my core.

In the morning I'm taken to urgent care and given a diagnosis of acute gastritis. A "straightforward" malady in which the lining of the stomach suddenly becomes inflamed, but of course I know, and Nivia knows, that nothing about this is straightforward. My body somehow absorbed the shock from yesterday in a way that bypassed my mind, and instead of having emotions, words, or thoughts, I have physical pain. I have a condition that can be named by a medical professional.

In the aftermath, I remain home from school for a week, during which time I let go of any desire to know more about my father. He becomes a shadow to me, a dark impression with no capacity for detail or depth. And as for the internet? It's clear it has everything. Even ghosts.

BLUE BUTTERFLY

We associate endangered species with epic, foreign landscapes shot in 4K resolution. We think of savannas shivering with pale green grasses, or rainforests gleaming in dappled light, but not more humble locations, like grocery store parking lots. American suburbs and their ecosystems of chain restaurants and civic centers do not immediately spring to mind, though of course, many of them contain their own brilliant matrix of life forms. A suburb of Los Angeles in fact is home to an extremely rare butterfly species, the *Euphilotes battoides allyni*, colloquially known as the El Segundo blue. The insect is less than three centimeters in length, and is, as the name suggests, blue—at least the males are. The females are tan, all the better to blend in with seacliff buckwheat, its only food source, which grows erratically at the city's western limits where it meets the beach. This area, full of industrial structures and Do Not Enter alcoves, prevents direct beach access, though remnants of its ecological past crack through, chiefly sand dunes, the buckwheat's preferred soil. Over a century ago, El Segundo was nothing but rolling sand dunes covered with this evergreen shrub, but as the municipality grew to encompass a Chevron oil refinery, an international airport, and a sewage treatment plant, the coastal area shrank, eventually resulting in the near disappearance of the butterfly. It has been on the US federal endangered species list since 1976.

Growing up, I was informed the butterfly was already extinct. Whether the adults around me were misinformed, or just pessimistic, hardly mattered. I never saw one, and no one I knew had ever seen one, and the way butterfly iconography was splashed all over town only further cemented the idea of extinction in my mind. In the same manner the profile of a bearded unicorn might be used for an investment-firm logo, the butterfly appeared as a graphic emblem on business cards and city banners, indicating something far more mythic than authentic, and eventually I forgot about it just as I forgot about griffins and the other wondrous creatures that populate childhood.

Swirling down into my current rabbit hole, the blue comes back to me. I'm googling a butterfly preserve in upstate New York, searching for its proprietor, and in the liminal state of scrolling and clicking, memories seep forward. I take a detour and open a new tab.

The internet says the butterfly is still with us thanks to the efforts of conservationists fostering buckwheat colonies. While still endangered, their numbers are increasing and an article claims you can see them fluttering around during their "flight season," which begins in late May and lasts throughout the summer.

IT'S A RIVER IN EGYPT

You hire a detective because you don't want to look at your own life.

LINK ROT

Link rot is an evocative term for something as simple as a 404 error. The invocation of "rot" produces images of mangled matter, of cattail reeds disintegrating into dark, black muck, which is more or less what is happening. On whatis.techtarget.com, link rot is defined as "the tendency of hypertext links from one website to another site to become useless as other sites cease to exist or remove or reorganize their web pages," which is a clunky way of saying "The number you have dialed is no longer in service." While links have been rotting since the birth of the web, in recent years the problem has surfaced as a lethal scourge.

To demonstrate the issue, researchers at Harvard Law School examined the hyperlinks in every *New York Times* article since its website's launch in 1996 until mid-2019. Within this period over two million links were identified with 72 percent of them categorized as "deep links," or hyperlinks to specific pages of websites (i.e., not home pages). Focusing on these deep links, the researchers discovered a whopping 25 percent of them were "dead." *The New York Times* was selected as the test case for this project because of its international reputation as a "standard-bearer for digital journalism, with a robust institutional archiving structure." The fact that a large portion of its outsourced material had evaporated from the planet was not viewed by the researchers as a "sign of neglect." Rather, it was interpreted as "a reflection of the state of modern online citation."

The repercussions of this state are, however, dire, particularly within the field of law. In March 2014 the *Harvard Law Review Forum* noted that "50% of the URLs within the US Supreme Court opinions suffer reference rot—meaning, again, that they do not produce the information originally cited."

In an article written for *The Atlantic,* Jonathan Zittrain, one of the Harvard researchers, states, "Sourcing is the glue that holds humanity's knowledge together." When a chain of references is interrupted or breaks, a specific channel of knowledge is permanently lost, and while this is problematic, the internet's purpose was never to hold steadfast or to archive. If it was built *to do* anything, it was to mutate.

VIRAL STRUCTURE

The simple efficiency of viral structure is breathtaking. Who knew it only took a shred of code enshrined in a protein shell to change lives? To wipe out chunks of civilizations? To break hearts?

ATHENA

"As far as I can tell, this is mankind's most honest
cognitive project. It is frank about the fact that all
the information we have about the world comes
straight out of our own heads, like Athena out of
Zeus's. People bring to Wikipedia everything they
know. . . . It has everything we know in it — every
thing, definition, event, and problem our brains
have worked on; we shall cite sources, provide links.
And so we will start to stitch together our version of
the world, be able to bundle up the globe in our own
story."

—*Flights* by OLGA TOKARCZUK,
trans. JENNIFER CROFT

ONLINE INVESTIGATOR SEARCH

The websites are exactly what you'd expect, peppered with iconic detective imagery from stock photo libraries and, in some cases, clip art collections. Most of them have that early-internet feel, with misaligned text and oddly sized graphics reminiscent of a time when one's vision couldn't easily be translated to screen. Googling "private detective services" feels like an archaeological expedition: it's one of the few searches that reveals the evolution of web design. Once you cut through a few superficial layers of results you will enter a realm where Comic Sans is a deliberate choice. It is a scary place, and even more frightening are sites for newer businesses that are still designed in that 1997 frame of mind. This leads me to suspect that either business turnaround is so incredible there's no time for branding, or that the webmasters are all of a certain age.

As I click through the results of "private detectives + Los Angeles" they seem to all share a similar constellation of elements:

- Silhouetted people
- Magnifying-glass pictures as logos, icons, or buttons
- Typefaces in bold colors ranging from neon green to bloodred
- Clip art of thumbprints, binoculars, and puzzle pieces—snapped in and out of place
- Photos of surveillance equipment, such as video camcorders and telephoto lenses
- A headshot of the main investigator, usually in black-and-white, and on occasion dressed as Philip Marlowe
- A pull quote with the number of years the investigator has been in "the biz"

I couldn't make up this shit if I tried.

CatchacheatPI.com, now seemingly defunct, used to focus on infidelity and offered an array of surveillance options from $350 to $2,199. Each package included a designated number of "tailing hours" and GPS data. Sunset Blvd. Investigations, still functioning, is more contemporary, advertising a combo of "21st Century Solutions" and "Old School Detective Skills." One of its specialties: background checks for internet dating services. Super Eye Investigations deals with locating deadbeat parents and other missing persons among a host of other services, including "electronic countermeasures." California Spy has a division devoted to the recovery of stolen artwork, and a tab on its site devoted to "P.I. Humor." (Potatoes make the best detectives. They always keep their eyes peeled. Etc.)

For kicks I run another search for London-based P.I.s and find a strange overlap of stock imagery: a firm on City Road features the exact same handsome, suit-clad "investigator" as a firm on Ventura Boulevard in Encino, California. The replication of the figure across space and time, and websites, can only mean one thing: there's a glitch in the matrix.

While mostly as atonal as their North American counterparts, there are fortunately no ex-coppers dressed as Sherlock Holmes. The Brits, as always, retain a measure of class, with the one exception of Shadow Private Investigators. Its site contains the Holy Grail of uncomfortable yet puzzling imagery:

- A perfectly impressed pink lipstick kiss on a man's shirt
- A white guy checking the cellphone of his Black girlfriend while she sleeps beside him in bed
- A close-up of a Nokia cellphone, circa 2001

- A man in a suit lying on his back in a field of yellow wild-flowers
- A satellite floating in outer space

None of this is encouraging.

I turn off my computer. My only real option is to ask some retired LAPD officer called Rusty for help, and I'm not sure if Rusty has it in him to find two dead people from the nineties. The closest service I can request from any of these detectives is "background check," or possibly "locate birth mother," neither of which suits my purposes. It seems easier to piece together a life from the 1850s, using whatever remnants of a paper trail and a locket photo, than a life from 1992, when digitization was still haphazard. The emphasis then was on preservation of truly old documents or the creation of new digital files from scratch. The documentation of the early to midnineties was strangely overlooked, as if it were too immediate for anyone to see. A whole segment of time was lost, and sure, major things were captured, but what about the everyday? What about the experience of the world the second before everything changed?

MONOLITH

A social network adapted from college "face books," or student directories, is launched in 2004. The Facebook, eventually just Facebook ("It's cleaner."), allows users to create profiles and "friend" other users on the site, creating vast webs of interconnection. A graphic representation of these connections appears on a user's profile, along with photos and basic information such as relationship status, hobbies, and interests. The later addition of a Wall feature provides space for users to post information that can then be "liked" by others in the user's network. This type of interaction constitutes a new form of social engagement. As the platform evolves, the history of a user's posts is formatted into a Timeline; the effect of scrolling through a person's online existence shifts Facebook away from an album or archival experience and toward one of presentation. Over time, messaging, games, classified ads, business profile pages, fundraising pages, and "stories" will be incorporated into the site, making it a monolith of digital life.

MEDICAL METAPHORS

An article titled "Using Metaphors in Medicine" begins,

> The language of medicine can be as clear as mud. A key reason for this is clinical medicine is not an exact science but more of a blended art form of science . . . set in a quagmire of human emotions and influenced by numerous abstract variables. Emotional experiences are notoriously difficult or impossible to convey by literal language. By using a metaphor to connect the relational pattern of a new experience with that of a familiar, emotion-laden one, we can create a contextual roadmap to understand and process a complex pattern of feelings. So in an attempt to find clarity and simplicity, patients and clinicians indulge in "medspeak" and metaphors when communicating about grave illnesses.

The notion of clinical medicine being a "blended art form" does not inspire a great deal of confidence until one realizes that human bodies are also a blend, or a "quagmire" of chemistry, experience, and emotion. This is perhaps why medicine favors the metaphorical framework Medicine-Is-War, which is by far the most pervasive metaphor within medical discourse, as physician Paul Hodgkin writes:

> The language that we use about our role as doctors is cast almost entirely by this metaphor and military images also appear in every aspect of medical language and jargon: It's an *overwhelming* infection; she's got an *infiltrating* carcinoma; the body's *defences*; he's having a heart *attack* . . .

Diseases also *invade* bodies, leave behind *victims,* and *destroy* cells. Hodgkin continues, "It is easier for doctors to bear the failure of medicine if the 'real' enemy is construed to be the disease." In this scenario, doctors assume the role of generals and treatment is weaponized, rendering the patient as little more than a battleground. The restoration of health acquires an aggressive tonality, which may or may not be useful for the healing process. The idea of "combating" an illness might destabilize a patient in a fragile state. The metaphor also places emphasis on the annihilation of the opponent/illness rather than on the state of the patient's health, which again may not be conducive to healing.

Closely tied with Medicine-Is-War is the Body-Is-a-Machine proposition, which transmutes illness into a system's malfunction. Medicine in this instance becomes engineering: worn-out joints are "upgraded," organs can be exchanged, and germs are malware, erratic pieces of code that require clinical removal. The allure of the mechanical metaphor eliminates the sloppiness of our biological reality, and makes it so every illness is but a problem to "troubleshoot," except bodies are a mess, the product of a billion years' worth of chaos and chance, and so solutions, if anything, are rare.

THE LITTLE ICE AGE

I am at a dinner party where a French girl is talking about the Little Ice Age, a weather phenomenon that struck Europe during the late fourteenth century. According to her, the plunge in temperature was caused by a series of volcanic eruptions; ash clouds congealed in the atmosphere and formed a thick shield across the sky. This caused glaciers to blossom like weeds, and the sun remained hidden for well over one hundred years. "People lived their lives in cold and darkness," she says, "and were sad." "Dejected," someone supplies from the end of the table. She nods solemnly and after a beat of heavy silence, during which she gives her Bakelite bangle a twist, she resumes in an almost sinister whisper, "The mood of the time was captured in works of art, you can see it in the paintings. There are no rays of light, no shine. Everything is this ice gray. The scenes of life have no joy. Lakes and rivers are shown frozen. The Thames froze over many times back then . . ."

We are a bric-a-brac collection, mostly lopsided artists and academics, curators, a programmer or two, and maybe even a shitty lawyer, approximating adulthood. The conversations revolve around the usual "grown-up" topics: the epic crawl toward the property ladder, down payments and what you have to do to get them together, cheap weekend breaks in former Soviet countries, craft beer, the failure of capitalism, and big talk surrounding what is most certainly imaginary culinary skill. The hosts tonight are celebrating the co-purchase of their flat with a mediocre five-course feast. Coffee tables of various heights have been linked together to create a banquet-style seating arrangement. Guests balance plates on palms and thighs to avoid bending over at sharp angles to eat, and wineglasses range from Turkish teacups to plastic champagne flutes. Somewhere a Spotify playlist pumps out Arcade Fire, and a few garlands of fairy lights fill in the rest of the décor.

Tonight is December 2 and there is a bite in the air that wasn't present two nights ago when it was still November. This is how we originally got onto the topic of the Little Ice Age. All of us had forgotten what it is to be cold, as we do every single year, and so we moved from the chill to the waning daylight to something I never could have seen coming. "Before this period of time there are very few depictions of winter in painting. Yes, yes really. Paintings began to show empty snow landscapes with tree skeletons. There are village scenes with peasants skating on ice, but the faces are hard. Lips are closed in straight lines." The French Girl pauses, flexes the muscles in her face, and draws a line in the air in front of her mouth.

"The psychological and environmental effects of the change were recorded in the paint. The canvases are evidence of this climate change, this tiny ice age."

Mostly everyone at the table presents as a headless torso, with faces only revealed if they happen to drift into a candle aura, which the French Girl now does deliberately, to dramatize her story. I worry, briefly, that her ponytail might catch fire. "The population suffered very much. There were many famines because nothing could grow, and then came the black death, which swept even more people away! Between the ice and the death, people didn't know what to do, so they began burning witches. They blamed witches, women really, for the spread of darkness."

"I'm so glad you said that," her American boyfriend violently interjects. "In my head, as you were talking, I kept chanting, 'Blame women, blame women, blame women.' It shows nothing has changed. We've blamed them for everything since the beginning of time—"

Then, to further sensationalize his point, the American Boyfriend puts his head near a flame. Just as his face materializes, I look over in his direction and get an immediate sick, horrible feeling that I've seen this guy's dick before—*not* like we've slept together or anything like that, but like I've seen him naked onstage or in a basement gallery, writhing away in a corner. The image of the white whale of his body with subcutaneous fat insulating his back and buttocks is vivid as can be, but I can't place it. The nakedness seems to have obliterated all other details of the encounter. While the rest of the guests march headfirst into the inevitable violence-against-women convo, I reach awkwardly for the untouched white wine, and then realize too late that I am now exposed. No sooner does this thought leave my mind than I feel the eyes of the American Boyfriend lock onto mine in some sort of questioning recognition. As he forcefully gestures through a list of moments the patriarchy has suppressed women's rights, he keeps the deepest and most hidden part of his black pupils narrowly fixed on mine while appearing to direct his exposition toward the entire table. To be clear: what's happening is not an intense sexual gaze, but something more fucked, like he wants to control how I think of him. The French Girl swoops back in, and through some heavy maneuvering, steers the conversation back to her point. "Some people realized that the witch burning did not restore heat and sun or drive the plague away, so they started to reject folklore and superstition. Out of all this came the Enlightenment, came science. You can trace a line from climate change to witch burning to science."

The tide of conversation gently goes out and drifts in another direction, though we all feel where it is going, because it's where every conversation goes these days. "That wouldn't be so bad, right? The end of everything?" says the girl on my right. "We deserve to undergo a mass extinction . . ."

A Swede a few seats down rolls a cigarette and makes motions to exit with it. I take the opportunity to also withdraw and meander to the bathroom. I shut the door behind me and lean into it. A line of moisture has formed on my upper lip, and I can feel a wave of heat rush up under my cheeks. I run the faucet and stick my face underneath it, rotating gently from left to right. After I dry off, I slump to the floor. It feels unreasonably good to sit. By the toilet I notice a lighter. I sweep it toward me with my foot. The queen is on it, grinning, in front of a Union Jack. I flick it a few times and watch the flame shudder and shift before settling into itself. Sooner or later, I'll have to go out there again. Later seems better.

Inside my blazer pocket I find an unwrapped stick of gum, an old tissue, and a crumpled receipt for a Pret A Manger salad I bought two weeks ago. I stand up and very neatly smooth out the creases of the receipt on the counter. Then I lift it to the ceiling, by the smoke detector, and light a corner on fire. As the paper catches and the flame eats away at it in a neat, red seam, I count very slowly from one to five, from five to ten, and when the screech of the alarm punctures the room tone, I drop the receipt in the toilet bowl and flush it away.

The living room is a tornado, with people reaching for jackets and scarves and purses and bags, limbs over limbs, pulling and stretching, getting tangled, trying to exit. There is a mad dash for the wine bottles on the table, and then, everyone is shoving into the corridor and down the stairs with more excitement than genuine concern. The American Boyfriend offers, "It is probably nothing, but since we just moved in, we should be careful!" The French Girl:

171

"I think it is a test! I remember the estate agent saying . . ." As the party reconfigures on the street, the neighbors also join in. The mood is bewildered, and in the jostling of bodies and phones and wine cups, I slide out into the night and disappear as quickly as possible.

VIVIAN'S BIRTH

Vivian was born weeks before her due date. Nivia, sensing something was wrong, took herself to the hospital, where she was promptly dismissed by the on-call physician. He told her that she was "imagining things," because, according to the calendar, "it wasn't time yet." So, she went home, closed the curtains, went to bed, and brought my mother into the world completely on her own.

OLDEST TRICK IN THE BOOK

If life has ever scraped you out and left you with no prospects, you can use art as a coping mechanism. You can apply it to your day-to-day. Take its content or its forms and use them to patch in what's missing. Take a fictional premise, maybe even a genre, and adapt it to your situation. See what happens.

DIGITAL FOOTPRINTS

The early 2000s were inundated with news items describing how the internet was "changing the face" of the fill-in-the-blank industry. These daily stories all had the same narrative: technology was rendering large segments of X industry irrelevant, and the internet was to blame. It was also responsible for the "disruption" of said industry's cornerstone values—such as journalistic integrity. Every imaginable sector was acknowledged to be in some way "degraded" by the dot-com—media, finance, retail, production, medicine, art, science, publishing, travel, education, the list went on. The only one never mentioned was private investigation, perhaps because tracing digital footprints was far easier than tracing physical ones, which meant, by extension: P.I. work just bled into normal life. Anyone could do it.

DO DO, DO DO DO DO

In 2005, YouTube, a video-sharing platform, makes its debut. YouTube allows users to "broadcast" themselves by uploading homemade content. They can also engage with the platform by commenting on, "liking," and "disliking" the work of other users. Initially conceptualized as a video dating site in the vein of Hot or Not, where "attractive" women were asked (via craigslist.org) to upload content of themselves in exchange for a one-hundred-dollar "reward," the site was forced to pivot when (unsurprisingly) it received no responses. Facing a lack of interest, YouTube broadened its content parameters. This eventually leads to the spread of iconic videos such as "Shoes" and "Gangnam Style." The most popular video of all time, uploaded on June 17, 2016, features two children singing a multi-verse ballad about a family of sharks' ill-fated hunting expedition. As of November 2, 2020, "Baby Shark Dance" has been viewed over eleven billion times, a number that outstrips the population of Earth by at least three billion.

THE 101 COFFEE SHOP

The joint sits on the corner of Franklin and Vista Del Mar right by the freeway overpass. It is a retro-style diner attached to a Best Western. Painted on the side of the motel is a giant mural of a coffee cup framed by the words LAST CAPPUCCINO BEFORE THE 101.

The inside is done up in a sixties style with all manner of browns, tans, and nudes coating the multitextured surfaces. Tile and faux rock make up the walls. The counter is laminate and long, stretching toward the back of the establishment in a thin wood-grain line. A strip of mirror, tipped at a curious angle, hangs above it, allowing customers in the vinyl swivel chairs below to spy on the customers in the booths behind them. Lights drop from the ceiling in translucent globes, hovering over the tables like small planets. In the glass case underneath the register are Butterfingers and York Peppermint Patties available for purchase, presumably for your road trip journey, and nearby, a plastic dome shields a lush chocolate cake from flies. Charm is well preserved. Almost twenty years old, the diner still feels like a secret. When it first opened, no one knew about it. You could come at any time of day and eat eggs, shrouded in an anonymous air. Then word of its late-night vegetarian offerings spread, and it became a Scene. Fortunately, the fever has since subsided, and its initial quiet has returned. Crowding however can still happen. This is Hollywood after all.

I slide into a booth, the Formica tabletop sticky with the residue of honey. There's a plastic squeeze bottle in the shape of a bear with its lid unscrewed. Evidence of a crime. The lighting is mercifully low and the jukebox plays The War on Drugs. Through the cutout window of the kitchen, I can see chef whites swiveling around and grilling something. A clock on the wall lets me know 2 A.M. is around the bend. When the waitress comes over in her Jetsons-like uniform dress, I order a coffee and a bagel, toasted dark. Her name tag says "Den." I briefly consider the reality of this as a name, and notice she's got a stroke of mascara curving out of her eye and slipping down her cheekbone. It could have only gotten there through the movement of tears, Kleenex, and clumsy reapplication. Her nose is red, either from cocaine or wiping sadness away, possibly both. She is incapable of eye contact during our exchange and when she walks away her gaze drills into the floor. I watch her punch my order into an iPad while hunching her shoulders around her ears. This girl, I know, is trying to disappear, and every so often she twitches, adjusting the collar or the cuffs of her uniform as if remembering she takes up physical space. She wipes down the counter in jagged strokes that form a cartoon mountain range, and then paces, checking her phone every few minutes. Something is or isn't happening.

I try to sharpen my mind for the drive down to Long Beach, thirty miles away. I stare straight ahead and rapidly blink a few times. I yawn, stretch my arms, but instead of focusing, my attention drifts dreamlike over an arrangement of plastic frames on the wall. They are solidly affixed to it but haphazardly spread, like salt grains brushed across a tablecloth. The frames contain photographs of different sizes and orientations. The era of them is hard to place and yet, the texture of the photo paper, the sun-warped color palette, and the poses of the subjects are immediately familiar. The picture closest to me is of a little girl dressed as a cowboy in denim overalls and a red bandanna. She rides a brown pony rigged to springs and shyly half smiles at the camera. This is a scene I've also starred in.

Another is a portrait of a kid with closed eyes and fingers crossed wishing into the air above flickering birthday candles. Sometimes it really does seem like all family photos are identical, the same five pictures taken over and over again throughout all of history. At the top of the wall are school portraits, glossy eight-by-tens showing soft young boys in front of paint-splattered backgrounds. They don't appear to be related, but here they are together on a diner wall. Farther down is a class photo. It is so sun bleached, the children look like ghosts dematerializing out of the marigolds and whites of the frame. These altered tones bleed into the photos surrounding it, affecting sunglasses, beach umbrellas, and vistas. Different decades become visible as I look closer, but just then my coffee arrives. Den the Waitress smacks it onto the table.

"Oh my god, I'm *so sorry*. I thought the table was, like, lower—"

"Don't worry about it, it's all fine," I tell her, pulling out a few napkins from the dispenser to cover the spill.

"Can I, here, let me top it up for you." And she flutters back to the counter to grab the pot.

The photos above the neighboring booth seem devoted to teenagers. There are prom pictures taken on front lawns and in front of trees, rosebushes, and swooping, polished banisters. An "alternative" couple, in leather jackets, leans against a vintage black Mustang. In another shot, a guy wears a Superman T-shirt underneath a dark blazer. He mimes tearing through the cotton while his date covers her mouth in awe, a wrist corsage blossoming from her lips.

"Here you are," Den says while carefully filling my mug and depositing my bagel in front of me.

"Are these pictures real?"

"What do you mean 'real'?"

"Like, do they belong to the owner, or did a designer buy them at flea markets?"

"Oh, I thought you meant, like, did someone do a casting and then photoshop them all to look old."

"No, I just mean do these people know they are on the wall of a restaurant?"

"They are friends of the owner—at least, that's what I read on the website. No one told me anything. But I never really thought of it like that before. Like, are all these people random and now in this place."

Her phone glows and shakes in her apron pocket and she vanishes in a puff of smoke.

Looking around I try to take in as many of the pictures as possible, but they start to recede. I see the frames link across the wall, forming a Tetris grid, but no longer the frozen scenes. My thoughts turn instead to the person who preserved these pictures. Not the people in them or the people who took them, but to the person who held on. Their installation in this unusual circumstance makes one thing very clear: it shows what it's like for a person to be moved. It shows the twisting of the heart that accompanies longing. It makes that motion *visible*. You can see it, filling in the space. The room is an album, spread open on one continuous plane.

I look down at my bagel and at nothing else until it is gone. At the register I pay and slip out the door without a second glance.

Outside, the night is motionless. The air, swollen with jasmine and some other plant scents, pins everything down. As I pass the edge of the motel, a voice says, "Do you have a light?"

It's Den, caught in the moonlight, with tears like little crystal fragments all over her face.

177

"Are you okay?"

"Yes. No. Not really. I'm sorry, do you have a light?"

"Yeah, just a sec."

I shuffle through my canvas sack and pass it to her, slightly confused because she seems the wrong age bracket for cigarettes, but what do I know? I notice her name tag seems to have had an E scraped off.

"Is your name actually Eden?"

"God no. It's Sarah. This belonged to the girl who had the job before me. All the customers kept asking me about it, so I just tried to change it somehow. I won't be here long, so I really haven't pushed to get my own."

The flame of the lighter washes out her face, makes it look like it belongs in one of the frames inside.

"Is this the Queen of England?" she says, flipping the lighter over and over.

"Yes."

"You've been to England?"

"Yeah. I live there actually."

"That is so incredible! I really want to go and see things in Europe . . ." She stops talking and we just stand there for a while, the smoke accumulating between us.

"Don't let it rewrite you."

"What?"

"The heartbreak. The boy. Your mom. Whatever it is. Don't let it change you . . . make you . . . bad."

She lets the cigarette go out and she attempts to light it again. I see her try to absorb what I've said, and when she gives the slightest impression of a nod, I walk away.

"Hey, wait—"

"It's yours."

I leave her near the corner and walk for what feels like hours to my car. In a second-floor apartment a window is open with the light on. A ripped young man washes dishes shirtless. On his head is a cowboy hat. A real one, with dust and worn edges, not a dinky prop you can buy in a store, and he is singing. His voice carries the deep swell of an Elvis imitation. The whole street is frozen except for this cowboy's sway and movements of a sponge. No dogs bark. No changes of light occur. The sounds of traffic are too far away to contaminate this residential strip. It is too early for birds. Too late for anyone normal, and not even the palm trees shiver. It's just me and this slow-motion mirage. I debate fumbling for my phone to record it, but somehow I know it will just evaporate if I do. The cowboy shuts off the faucet and does a little pirouette with a hand towel before hanging it on a hook. And people tell me they hate this town.

PROCEDURE?

Can history be biopsied? Can a person—like the French Girl—really drop a needle into time and extract a coherent narrative from the sample? Isn't it, after all, the structure of the needle that forces tissue, or elements, into a readable line?

PHOTO OF NIVIA IN A FIELD

There is a photograph of Nivia in a field wearing a dress with a scalloped neckline. Her hair is draped over one shoulder, and she uses a ribbon as a headband. In the distance are rows of tropical plants with fronds spread out like hands. The earth where she stands barefoot is dry and dusty. Awkwardly balanced on her hip is her daughter as a delightfully pudgy baby. By contrast, Nivia's arms look like twigs. Bones are visible everywhere on her and despite the fact that there are no objects in the foreground to give a sense of scale, you can tell she is a tiny, delicate woman. It seems improbable that she is holding a baby, let alone produced one, yet she is incandescent. Her eyes blaze into the camera, burning the film inside it.

TOTALLY ACCEPTABLE

"A form of private investigation is today a normal part of life for many people, given the advent of the Internet generally, and social networking in particular. An acceptable kind of voyeurism is sanctioned by Google or Facebook, as we peer into the private lives and spaces of others — places which once, not so long ago, were guarded as private, intimate, secret. In return we show a willingness to exhibit our own private experience for public consumption — through Facebook, Twitter, other online platforms and reality television, all mechanisms set up to enable individuals to *display* their private selves and activities."

— *The Private Eye: Detectives in the Movies* by BRAN NICOL

VIRAL SENSATION

Many people long to become A Sensation, but it is only by exhibiting viral characteristics that they can infiltrate public consciousness with any significant effect. We might ask why this is happening. Why does a vast sector of humanity aspire to become *a feeling* and diffuse? Is it for the usual motivations: fame, love, or money? Transcendence of the ordinary? Perhaps it is something less obvious. What if it's simply a longing to be envied? Not desired, not adored, but hate-loved? Idolized, and yet also abhorred—for if people feel this unnatural combination of emotions about you then surely you must *mean something*. If you infect people and their response to you is fevered, involving a gag, a cringe, or a hurl, you've created a sensation—which is power. Except, it's not power in the traditional sense of "power move" or influence. It is something quite different. If you exchange your corporeality to hover, cloudlike, in the minds of others, you lose time, which is to say: mortality. The power is the decision to exist, like the virus, in a ceaseless loop of replication where birth and death are rendered irrelevant.

LADY X

A friend texted a link to an article published in her college alumni magazine. It was a profile of a female private investigator who sounded extremely intelligent, and not without empathy. Her Squarespace website was vague, but not tacky, and featured a thumbprint icon so abstracted it could easily be mistaken for a pleasant graphic. I made note of the phone number on the contact page.

The first time I called, her salutation hit me like a face slap. The tone was so abrasive it stung, and it summoned the image of an aggro mom tossing her two sweaty, hyperactive brats into the back seat of a van after football practice. "HELLO," she spat into the phone. As I swallowed and prepared to issue a hello back, I caught the screech of an engine in the background, and instinctively hung up.

Ten days later I tried again. The greeting was identical.

"HELLO."

"Hi, um, is this Lady X?"

"YES."

"Hi. Okay. A friend of mine was in your class at UNIVERSITY—"

"You read the article."

I prattled on about the magazine and the profile, and then awkwardly transitioned into the reason for my call: would she investigate my dead parents? I wanted her to fill in the black holes of their timelines with information that might seem basic but would mean the world to me. I needed to know where they worked, and for how long, and did they owe anyone money? Where else in LA did they live? I needed to know about David and his controversial beliefs, and if possible, when and how HIV entered the picture.

This all came out in one long ribbon that became increasingly tangled the longer I spoke. I hoped she would detect I was struggling and would kindly commandeer the conversation back to a target, as any normal person might, but her end of the line remained silent. Unfortunately, my only recourse was to continue awkwardly babbling until she finally interrupted me.

"This sounds more like a local ancestry project."

"Oh. Okay."

"What I do is, someone calls me up and says a guy fled child support or bail, someone disappears and someone needs them, right? So I sift through data and I form a digital trail of that person. I can get anecdotes from firsthand accounts, I go on Facebook, but all of it is current, is happening right now. It's a different ball game. If this was fifteen years ago I could trace a person's MySpace page and see they were part of such and such a group and then track down people that way . . . but you're talking thirty-five to forty years ago, this little crevice of time before any recent history was extensively digitized."

"Right."

"If I were you I'd go to the library, visit city hall, pull voter registration cards. I would talk to people who knew them. Find out where they used to live and talk to neighbors and get anecdotal stuff—that's what's going to be of interest to you anyway. Talk to your family, get addresses of places they used to work. Oh—and check local newspapers. See if they were mentioned in 5K results or if they coached little league . . ."

I stopped listening. Her assumption that there were friends and family left to speak to implied, at least to me, that she was probably shit at her job. If any of this were an option, why would I call her? I just wish Lady X had openly said, "You are wasting my time," but I don't even remember how the conversation ended.

PERSECUTED DOCUMENTS

A website specializing in data dumps or "leaks" of classified information appears in 2006. The stated aim of the site, WikiLeaks, is to expose restricted materials pertaining to "war, spying and corruption" to the public eye. Its founder, the mercurial Julian Assange, later describes the project as "a giant library of the world's most persecuted documents." Not without controversy, WikiLeaks will unearth profound ethical considerations right alongside highly sensitive video, private correspondences, and memos.

INCESSANT MOVEMENT

It always starts with something piercing the heart. Nothing as glamorous or succinct as an arrow, but something unfinished, like a shard of glass. You can't see it or put a name to it. At best you can sheepishly refer to it as a "yearning," which is much deeper than longing and more complex than pining. To yearn for something is to have desire leak through you and pull you forward in a way that your steps are not your own and your thoughts are not your own. When your life aches for something you can't put your finger on, the only recourse is incessant movement. Your only recourse is a quest.

PEOPLE REMEMBER DIFFERENTLY
THAN THEY USED TO

People remember differently than they used to. We don't remember things the way our parents or our grandparents did. We curate the remembrance of an event as the event is occurring. We construct memory while embedded inside an experience, meaning the future is already happening when we are dancing at a concert or laughing at a birthday party. We create the future as it erupts in the present, and later that same future will emerge in a different present, as part of the present moment, but as the past, as memory, when a post is tapped on or scrolled through. All of these posts, all of these recorded documents, show a sprawling network of curated remembrances, but what of the actual experience? Did something even happen if it was constantly being shaped for another time and place?

There is probably a generational shift every decade, with the communication of memory, and its documentation, but now, how long is a generation?

POSTCARD, 2013

My phone rings. It's Nola.

"What are you doing right now?"

"Nothing."

"Be downstairs in five."

This is a thing we do, me and Nola. She is my only friend with a car, and really, my only friend, so when San Francisco starts to feel too damp and spread out one of us calls the other and we drive. She pulls round to the front of my building and then we fly down Geary to the beach where we disappear into sheets of fog. Sometimes we do this late-night, other times when the day is slipping off the sky and everything turns translucent. Usually, we meet when all the good people of the world are settling into their evening activities— cooking, dog walking, dinner with the fam, or primping for a night on the town. We are not those people.

The time it takes Nola to leave her apartment and get to mine is precisely the same amount of time it takes me to grab my bag, hop in the elevator, ride down five floors, and exit the lobby by theatrically throwing open the doors like a silver-screen siren.

"Hey, girl."

"Hey."

I slide into the passenger seat, buckle up, slip my hood off my head. She reaches over and turns up the radio. Tonight I can tell we won't say much. It's Friday and: we're exhausted. We don't need to talk about it. She and I have the same dull feeling pressing against our skulls. During the week it downshifts into background noise, diffusing through obligations and responsibilities, but once everything calls it quits the feeling returns. In our case we are afflicted with a condition no one likes to discuss but that is common among young women: the utter misery caused by the unbridled desire for sex and the total lack of anyone suitable to get it on with. Symptoms consist of flesh rotting off the bones and slithering into a puddle during what is considered the patient's "prime." There is no cure unless you are willing to abandon your standards—which everyone does in the end, but then you have to live with the fact that you've abandoned your standards. As Nivia would say, in a mangled approximation of god knows what proverb, "You can't win by losing."

It is a cool fifty-two degrees according to the dashboard display and the fog unfurls its limbs into the narrow cavities between buildings. The peaks and valleys of the city provoke the mists of the Pacific into supernatural action, and it gets inside your joints, filling them with clouds.

On this side of town, after midnight, the streets are still, but tonight feels empty in a particularly surreal way: a tumbleweed could pass us right now and it wouldn't be out of place. As if to accentuate this vibe, all the chandeliers in the Lamps Plus storefront extinguish simultaneously, then the signal changes, and Nola floors it. I roll down the windows and our hair whips around us in sharp angles. The road rises and we glide over the small hills, which increase in amplitude as the neighborhoods change. At the top of Twenty-sixth Avenue, the green and gold onion domes of the Holy Virgin Russian Orthodox Cathedral sprout out of a boring block of banks and office-supply stores. The tagline of the church, JOY OF ALL WHO SORROW, is emblazoned on a changeable letter marquee. Inside there is a relic, one of the few to make it to this side of the Pacific.

I imagine the withered limb of a saint waiting quietly in the dark for sunrise.

Then it's just Sleep Train Mattress Centers, karate dojos, and basketball courts for miles. They turn into streaks in my peripheral vision, and then the streaks gradually morph into two-story Marina-style homes dipped in eggshell and rose, most of them dark except for a porch light here and there. One has a group of people illuminated in a bay window. They are laughing and swirling long-stemmed glasses of wine. I think I hear Nola sigh. On the radio, "Bitch, Don't Kill My Vibe" comes on. She turns it up and the bass moves beneath us. The jagged ruins of the Sutro Baths come into view, their concrete fragments tearing up the night like prehistoric teeth. Families once swam here under vaulted glass ceilings. They took trolley cars from deep within the city and crossed sand dunes to get here. Adolph Sutro, with a type of consideration absent in most other mayors, built out the public transit system so citizens could access his attraction, but then it caught fire and burned to the ground. The land still draws visitors. I've seen marriage ceremonies at sunset on the cliffs, and teenagers doing drugs in the caves. Tourists come and take photographs, then dare one another to hop across the algae-infested pools.

We surge down the hill and pass the Cliff House hanging over the sea. I imagine the crisp white napkins and water glasses set out for tomorrow's brunch already collecting dust. The original Cliff House, built in 1858, was made of wood harvested from a shipwreck up the coast. Traces of that event must have lingered in those "reclaimed" logs, as the restaurant was rebuilt shortly after its inception, and then three times more. There is a well-known photograph of one of its incarnations, Victorian in style, getting struck by a razor-thin blade of lightning.

The Great Highway shuttles us forward, beyond the Dutch windmills of Golden Gate Park, the glowing Safeway on La Playa, and the Beach Chalet, and after a few more turns we dead-end into Ocean Beach. Tall mounds of sand surround the parking lot and beach wood logs act as demarcation devices. Somewhere out in front of us is the sea. The magnetism of its currents registers on the lower, subconscious frequencies and pulls us in.

Nola shuts off the engine and puts her feet, clad in some UGG knockoffs, on the dash. Everything settles and we look at nothing. After a few moments, Nola turns the car back on and rolls down the back windows. The waves come in.

"I went out with Mike again last night," she says.

"Oh yeah?"

Mike is a nice guy. I don't know him well but he seems, you know, not like a douchebag. They met at a party. He was the cater waiter running the bar. Under normal circumstances Nola would never have slipped him her number but times are tough. Over the last few months they have seen each other here and there. He thinks she's "cool." He told me this during the one and only conversation he's bothered to have with me. It lasted two minutes.

"He took me to Tacolicious in the Marina. Then we went to Romolo for drinks after. It was . . . nice . . ."

"So, boring as fuck, in other words."

"But he treats me like I matter . . . sort of."

"How many times have you been out now?"

"Like eight or nine."

"In three months?"

"Something like that."

We go back to listening to the waves. I let the surf lull all the dumb shit out of my brain and what remains are trolley cars winding across sand dunes in 1890, taking people to the edge of the sea through the terrain we've just driven. I feel them there, under us, somehow still moving, still living. San Francisco is like this, the ghosts never really leave, but stay on forever, reenacting some type of gold rush bust and boom cycle. I briefly see the Cliff House pierced by a liquid line of light, its turrets punctured by a seething, elemental force. Eventually I ask, "What are you going to do?"

"I don't know" is all she can say.

I start to braid my hair in a rope and pretend I can see through the blackness in front of us all the way to Japan.

"You know what I dislike the most?"

"I can't even begin to imagine. His job? His taste in movies? How he mistakes vigor and pressure for artistry when he's massaging your clit?"

"He wore a Star Wars T-shirt out last night."

"I'm sorry?"

"I mean, it wasn't exactly a Star Wars T-shirt."

"Nola, what the fuck do you mean? 'It wasn't exactly a T-shirt?' "

"No—it was a T-shirt, but it had a stormtrooper on it . . . holding a surfboard on a beach. The *point* is: he wore a fucking T-shirt on our date and I wore a tiny little dress with spaghetti straps in the freezing, forty-degree night to look hot as fuck. I wanted to dress up, get my tits out for a change, ditch this pathetic North Face fleece I wear every single night. Get out of these disgusting UGGs." She kicks a leg off the dashboard, then puts it back down elegantly. "I was just like: do you want me to blow you tonight or not? Wear a goddamn shirt with buttons on it then, for christsake—at least until we are dating for real, or an actual thing, or are married—or whatever the fuck."

"Was it a drawing of a stormtrooper?"

"No. A photograph."

"Was it in color?"

"Jesus, Heather, that's your takeaway?"

Two whole minutes go by.

"Black-and-white. It was a black-and-white photograph."

"Okay, he obviously could have put a little more effort into his appearance knowing that you'd probably be all dolled up and have sex with him but the truth is, you just don't like him."

"But he's nice."

"But you're bored."

I grab a woolly IKEA blanket from the back seat and tuck it around my legs. I have never had Nola's problem. I have never been with someone I was lukewarm about in order to pass the time, mostly because my feelings are polarizing: I either really like a guy or I don't, and if I don't there is not enough alcohol in the entire universe that will make him attractive to me. So, my problem is I'm alone way too much, and her problem is she's with too many guys she's only "meh" about. Or, if you looked at all this from a different angle you could say we actually have the same problem: if nothing sparks the heart, how do you know it's still there? You don't, and the continued absence of electrical activity will shred a person down to smithereens.

"This is more romantic than anything I've done with Mike."

"Sitting and freezing to death in a car?"

"No. Looking out at an ocean vista on a moonless night while listening to the waves."

"Are you fucking kidding me? We can't see a damn thing out there!"

She gets out her phone and takes a photo of our beautiful scenic view, and cackles, throwing her head back. The sound of her laughter cracks the gravity lodged in the car.

"Something to remember this moment by!"

"Forever and ever!" I shout. Then I lean my body out the window and shout into the wind like I'm in a teen flick from 1998, "Forever and ever, world! Don't you forget us!"

We drive back home, slower now. At the transition point between neighborhoods, on Twenty-ninth Avenue, all the frenetic energy of "Frisco" crawls back under our skin and stays there, twitching. We don't belong here, but we don't know where else to go.

I turn the radio on. By miracle, we find "Get Ur Freak On" and begin a full-on improvised dance routine. My shoulders shrug and twist themselves in figure eights. Nola points finger guns at invisible targets over the steering wheel. Our hips shake from side to side. I bend over and switch my kneecaps flapper style. She fist pumps the air. For two and a half minutes we are the happiest girls in the universe. Shimmering. Invincible. And then the song ends.

We pull into the yellow zone in front of my building. I lift my fog-filled skeleton from the seat and get out. Before I close the door I say, "Send me the beach photo?"

"Sure, as soon as I get home."

"Cool."

"And then, ten years from now, I'll print it out and send it to you as an actual postcard that says 'Wish You Were Here.'"

Stepping into my elevator that smells of disinfectant and moo shu pork, I think of how much I love Nola and how, if she remembers the postcard in ten years' time, she would be, without question, my Most Favorite Person Ever. But of course, in ten years' time she'll be married to a guy like Mike, or maybe even Mike himself if things pan out, and she won't think twice about these drives down the coast where we tried to erase our loneliness.

I open my apartment door while these thoughts slip into one another. I put my keys on the ledge, the old wall fixture designed for a telephone. "Hello, house," I call out into the dark. The refrigerator buzzes against the tile floor in the kitchen. Other than that, it's quiet.

TAXONOMY

"I'd like to share a revelation that I've had during my time here. It came to me when I tried to classify your species. I realized that you're not actually mammals. Every mammal on this planet instinctively develops a natural equilibrium with the surrounding environment, but you humans do not. You move to an area and you multiply and multiply until every natural resource is consumed and the only way you can survive is to spread to another area. There is another organism on this planet that follows the same pattern. Do you know what it is? A virus. Human beings are a disease, a cancer of this planet. You are a plague, and we are the cure."

— AGENT SMITH, *The Matrix*

AMSLER GRID

Nivia kept copies of the Amsler grid in all rooms of our house. They were affixed to the refrigerator with souvenir magnets from tourist-trap cities, and stuck onto doors with Scotch Tape. The "original" was issued by her UCLA ophthalmologist, and its duplicates were made on the library photocopier as well as Vivian's old fax machine. The fax versions had short life spans; the grids would smear off the smooth, thin paper, and the edges of the resultant prints were also perpetually curling, trying to resume the scrolled form they originated from.

Over time, every single grid became defective, worn out from time or light, or the occasional leak. However, none of them were ever removed, even long after Nivia's condition had solidified into blindness. Somehow, I never found this strange, the continued presence of what amounted to a useless geometry peppering our walls. I just accepted their permanence, though I cannot say if this was the same for Nivia. She may have grown so accustomed to them that they ceased to produce any effect on her consciousness. Alternatively, the grids might have meant a great deal to her. It could be these feeble paper charts offered an iota of continuity in a household that made no sense, their lines extending off the page and connecting together throughout the space, forming a lattice, a net that could hold us.

A SHORT BURST OF INCONSEQUENTIAL INFORMATION

In 2006, a "microblogging" site called Twitter emerges. Essentially a chimera of SMS-style messaging and a social media network, users formulate content within 140-character transmissions called "tweets." The word "twitter," defined as "a short burst of inconsequential information," perfectly encapsulates the initial, inane novelty of the platform, but within three years Twitter morphs from a communication tool focused on status updates to a credible news source capable of disseminating information at unprecedented speeds. This evolution from trivial to vital unsettles the balance of the social media ecosystem within human life.

LEEUWENHOEK

Antonie van Leeuwenhoek, the "father of microbiology," had no background in science. He was not a member of the aristocracy and had no university degree of any kind. Born in Delft in 1632, the only language he spoke was Dutch, and sources stress the fact that it was a "low Dutch." At fourteen, he tried to learn the law from his uncle, but it didn't take. Before that, his fate had most likely been sealed as a basket maker, as his father was a basket maker and all his relatives on that side of the family were basket makers . . . but when he was six his father died, disrupting the course of things, and establishing a bizarre precedent of loss in his life: Leeuwenhoek endured the deaths of his stepfather, first wife, four children, and second wife, but lived to the ripe old age of ninety at a time when life expectancy rarely surpassed forty. After the law debacle, Leeuwenhoek moved to Amsterdam, where he apprenticed under Scottish haberdasher William Davidson for six years. It was during this time that Leeuwenhoek was first exposed to lenses. "Glass pearls" were tools of the textile trade used to determine the quality of fabric. Like jeweler's loupes, they sat directly in the eye socket, setting the activity of observation within the intimate realm of the face.

In 1654 Leeuwenhoek returned to Delft and established his own haberdashery. He also, perhaps idiosyncratically, assumed a variety of public service roles including surveyor, chamberlain, and "official wine-gauger." This demonstrated an enterprising, if not ambitious, spirit. Case in point, he began forging and grinding lenses in the back room of his shop. Mining his personal experience with glass pearls, Leeuwenhoek created a delicate globule from a thread of soda lime glass that was nearly three hundred times more powerful than the popular disk-shaped lenses used in the microscopes of the day. However, due to its size and shape, the globule was unsuitable for use within a conventional microscope, so Leeuwenhoek constructed a device that a viewer could hold right up to the eye, not unlike a Venetian mask. It was unusual and yet wholly superior to the models made famous by Galileo and Robert Hooke, which invited viewers to look downward at a specimen through a tube. Presumably, Leeuwenhoek began his lens and microscope explorations as a part of his professional endeavors, but then he did something wholly unexpected: he turned his creation to the natural world.

There is no account of or explanation for why Leeuwenhoek ventured down this path, though a quote from a letter written in his twilight years provides some insight: "My work, which I've done for a long time, was not pursued in order to gain the praise I now enjoy, but chiefly from a craving after knowledge, which I notice resides in me more than in most other men." This craving led him to examine red blood cells, wood grain, muscle fibers, algae, sperm, vessels of pig brains, and bee stingers under his lens. He then documented these findings in meticulous illustrations and copious notes, which were later shared with the Royal Society in London at the urging of his friend, decorated physician Regnier de Graaf.

With the encouragement of the Society, Leeuwenhoek fashioned more lenses, built more microscopes, and obsessively investigated the material of nature. In a drop of rainwater, he discovered "animalcules," or "little animals," swimming of their own accord. This would prove to be a groundbreaking observation. The existence of life beyond the range of human vision was unfathomable in the seventeenth century. Like heliocentrism before it, the idea of a micro-

195

scopic reality created an existential threat to man's position in the universe, so while Leeuwenhoek was completely mesmerized by the self-propelled movements of his single-celled organisms (or proto-zoa, as they would later be identified), his heart sank. This discovery, he knew, would have a profoundly damaging effect on his reputation, and yet he reported it anyway. Consequently, when the Royal Society received his findings, they did not hesitate to label him a charlatan despite the incredible accuracy of all his previous work. The matter was only resolved when Leeuwenhoek arranged for a group of religious leaders to visit his workshop and observe the animalcules firsthand.

The episode, surprisingly, left no mark on Leeuwenhoek, and he pursued study of the microscopic realm for the next fifty years, submitting reports to the Royal Society up until the week he died. Each submission chronicled a sight never before witnessed by a human being.

This story, quite literally, is about vision, but not in the obvious sense; it's about space breaking down, condensing, and folding up into some entirely new experience that could be held straight in the retina.

EMERGENT BEHAVIOR

"Some of the more convincing evidence for internet consciousness might be difficult to perceive, since we ourselves would be the nodes and neurons that constitute the brain. For some social scientists, the many political movements that have originated on social networks qualify as 'emergent' behavior—

phenomena that cannot be attributed to any one
person, but belong to the system as a whole."
— "Is the Internet Conscious? If It
Were, How Would We Know?"
by Meghan O'Gieblyn

FINDING THE P.I.

After I hung up with Lady X, I experienced a single and precise moment of levity, as if a heavy backpack had just slid off my spine. I felt
my scapula float away and drift off into space, and the habitual,
crushing tension around my neck suddenly vanished. I felt the actual motion of something leave me, and in that I realized just how
gone my parents were. The weightlessness ceased. I returned to
earth. What little paper evidence there was of their existence would
be near impossible for a Luddite like me to obtain. There wasn't a
professional around who was going to help me with this, other than
a shrink, and that was debatable. I once saw a therapist who told me
my emotional logic was akin to the "magical thinking of children."
A few weeks later, after this "revelation," I broke down in her office
and sobbed for ten minutes straight. Once I had collected myself,
she looked straight into my eyes and said, "You are terrifying when
you cry," as if this information would somehow be beneficial to
me. Between the magic and the terror, who knows when the healing was supposed to begin.

I knew if I wanted information about my parents, it was likely I'd
have to find it solo. I also knew, unequivocally, that this would kill
me. I did not want to go search for things. Inevitably, this would
involve the internet and I had already experienced the piercing

shock of what it could offer. What I envisioned was hiring a third party to serve as a filtration device, someone who could mine the available data and then present it in a sanitized report, scrubbed free of misinformation or exaggeration. This way, the dirty work might be avoided, and I might have a chance to actually process what any of this meant.

For several weeks I did nothing, then one afternoon I stumbled into an art gallery. The show was like a poetic history pamphlet whose panels had been severed and spread across multiple rooms. Roving through it felt like floating through an information sea of hair barrettes, chunks of text, sewing tools, and translucent airmail envelopes. The artist had reconstituted the lives of her Polish grandparents through ephemera. Details of recovered documents, such as property division lines and signatures, were photographed in close-up. These images were then converted into long, rectangular textiles that hung heavily across the walls. The way they were arranged somehow evoked the quintessential cartoon treasure map with tiny, dotted lines linking symbols across unbound space. Walking from room to room my feet seemed to create their own trail connecting things, like an embroidered rose on a handkerchief to a diary entry. I spent a long time with a simple porcelain teacup rimmed with gold, and over the course of those minutes, a bolt of lightning struck my skull. It dawned on me that I might form my "case" in terms of "artistic research" and recruit help through unconventional channels.

Artistic research is an emergent discipline that involves an open marriage between the academic and the creative. It is predicated on the rigor of academia but tangos with the free and easy je ne sais quoi of contemporary art. Artists who bill their work as "artistic research" tend to do so because what they produce is often weak visually and thus needs "concepts" to prop it up. Other times they might harbor secret desires to be a part of the scholastic realm but lack the spine to play by its rules. The result is often an indeterminate mishmash in which the aesthetic or visual component of art is abandoned, despite art being a form predicated on optical engagement (sound art exempt). The sloppiness of this discipline has always been a source of irritation, but it occurred to me then that sloppiness is perhaps exactly what I needed. So: why not give it a try?

CATERPILLAR VIRUS

A friend of mine is spending the night on my bedroom floor, nearly underneath the coffee table. We are both reading, waiting to board that train to slumberland, when she says, "Did you know caterpillars liquefy their organs in their cocoons? It, like, comes down with a virus that turns its body into a soup."

"And the soup turns into a butterfly?"

"Yeah."

"And a virus turns the caterpillar into a soup?"

"Yeah."

"Where did you find out about this?"

She struggles to hold up an oversized glossy, a culture-fashion hybrid in which writers inject their socially conscious work with sex and cultural theory. The article, she goes on to say, is about the use of social media in revolutions, and somehow the butterfly-caterpillar-virus is symbolic of all that.

A few days later, I look up "caterpillar cocoon virus." The caterpillar, as it turns out, does liquefy itself. There is a moment when you could slice open a cocoon and the former caterpillar would ooze out, but this is caused by an enzyme and not a virus. The caterpillar digests itself, leaving behind clusters of highly specialized cells known as imaginal discs that contain the blueprint data for the butterfly's new body. These cell discs draw on the nutrient-rich soup of the former caterpillar and, over time, wings, antennae, and a mouth, coiled up like a French horn, develop.

The distinction between a virus and an enzyme for the general public probably doesn't mean anything—it certainly doesn't for the caterpillar. All it knows is that it must dissolve to move forward.

THE BERLIN PATIENT

At the 2008 Conference on Retroviruses and Opportunistic Infections held in Boston, Massachusetts, the anomalous case of the "Berlin Patient" is presented. The patient, a forty-year-old American man living in Berlin, was cured of HIV while undergoing intensive treatment for acute myeloid leukemia. After receiving chemotherapy, the patient required a bone marrow transplant to rebuild his decimated immune system. The bone marrow came from a donor with a rare genetic mutation that confers resistance to HIV. This trait was essentially "passed on" to the patient through the transplant, and over time he reached HIV-negative status. While technically a scientific victory, the experience of the cancer and the treatment was nearly unbearable for the patient, who had to undergo the transplantation twice; the first time only annihilated the HIV, leaving the cancer intact. The patient endured paralysis, temporary blindness, and delirium, and was eventually placed in a medically induced coma to recover, making this situation a onetime occurrence rather than a strategy for universal treatment.

NET

If you google "net," you have to filter through net worth, net income, Netflix, net neutrality, and Net-A-Porter to get anywhere near the actual object. A net, as a noun, is so basic it hardly seems worth mentioning, except it is a structure repeated throughout the known world: spiderwebs, curtain mesh, graph paper, the veins of plant leaves, the Lambert azimuthal projection, the arrangement of nerves in a jellyfish. Even gravity is visually represented as a grid of interconnected lines that warp and curve around celestial bodies like giant fishnets. A net, a lattice, a web, and a grid are all interchangeable terms for the form of one thing linked to another via a tie, knot, or node, and so more than being an object or structure, a net is a situation: it is a relationship of links that incites connectivity, like thousands of tree roots mingling miles beneath the forest floor, or a person. A person is also a situation, one that transmits, conducts, and links to other systems.

PENGUIN MAN

I click on a video in my Facebook feed. It's about an old man in Brazil who rescued a baby penguin on the beach outside his home. The penguin was covered in oil and other toxic debris, so the man took it home, cleaned it up, and nursed it back to health for ten days. On the eleventh, he brought the penguin back to the ocean and attempted to release it into the wild, but it did not want to go. The man kept trying and the penguin kept staying, and it lived with the man for the next several months before vanishing into its little aquatic life. What makes the story so extraordinary is that the penguin returns to visit the man each year. The video captures one of their reunions: the penguin is ecstatic, bounces around, wags its tail, and flaps its wings at the old man. The old man in turn weeps, smiles, and takes the penguin into his arms like a long-lost friend.

Watching the video, something happens to me. A feeling, which seems to have no real contextual basis, rises like mist from some deep interior space. I try to pin it on the weathered nature of the man's visage, encrusted with lines, and on the creature itself, but I know it's a ruse. Whatever this feeling is, it is not a reaction to witnessing this otherworldly relationship but has been there all along. This chemistry of images simply unlocked it. Again, I watch the wing flaps, the tears, the embrace, and suddenly I have the thought: maybe it is possible to wander the face of the Earth for a lifetime and finally, toward the end of it, have something, just one thing, make sense.

FAINTING

I lied earlier when I said I couldn't elicit my relationship with Nivia within the space of a single scene. There is in fact one that captures the intricacies of our dynamic:

Home from university with the flu I curl up in bed shivering. Glued inside a hoodie and all manner of sweats I can't seem to retain any heat. My white MacBook, balanced precariously on the edge of the bed, is playing episodes of *Sex and the City*. I had tried reading but the letters wove out of their words and floated around the page, so I gave in to binging instead. The show comes at me as a moving magazine, with editorial spreads enlivened by multiple frames per second. The pictures glide by with punch lines and engulf me within a tulle-and-chiffon reality until Nivia comes in to tell me lunch is ready. I hit the space bar.

"I'm not feeling well enough to eat."

"You have to eat," she says from the doorway. "You have to give your body strength so you can go back to school."

"I don't think I can sit up. Can you bring it in here?"

"No. You have to eat at the table."

She leaves the room, an invisible vacuum sucking her back into the kitchen, leaving an ominous void in the doorway. Something is not right. When I have been ill in the past Nivia restricted my activities in accordance with some Victorian-era conception of wellness; at the first sign of a sniffle, I was always rushed to a doctor, and then consigned to bed rest without privileges, not even that of a shower, for fear that wet hair might exacerbate my symptoms. Going outside was inconceivable, so the sudden enforcement of table dining is frankly baffling.

I take a moment to suss out the location of my limbs. After finding all four of them I judge whether they can take me anywhere. It seems unlikely so I resume watching Charlotte tell Harry he needs a back wax so they can publicly lounge poolside in the Hamptons. A few minutes later, Nivia reappears.

"Why aren't you at the table?"

"Grandma, I just don't think I can move."

"That's nonsense."

She does not move and does not speak, so I take this to mean that I should move and speak, but instead I ooze, amoeba-like, out from the covers. The next thing I know, I'm at the table with no memory of how I've arrived. Lines of sweat drip down my face and intermingle with one another. I focus on holding my body upright without swaying. Soup arrives. I try to get a few swallows in, but I can feel them not wanting to stay down. I try to apologize but then I see the glistening points of light form inside my field of vision. I become distracted by them, then enamored, shocked to find how accurately the expression "seeing stars" describes what I am experiencing. I stand up and head for the bedroom or the toilet, anywhere that isn't here. I get the feeling I am being yelled at, but the sounds are so distant I can't make much sense of them, and for once I don't care. I allow myself to disobey and feel delightful. Glee inflates my joints and in fact, I am floating, levitating off the ground, gliding to the corridor as everything dims.

I wake up on the laminate floor flat on my stomach. My head is cocked at a strange angle, and my mouth is open, a thread of drool coming out of it. I search my brain for my last memory and slowly piece together that I have fainted. The strange euphoria that precipitated it whispers back through me, the feeling of being carried away . . . Nivia, still talking, hoists me up like a marionette. She threads her upper body under one of my arms, and through sheer brute force, reestablishes my verticality. We shuffle toward the bedroom like this, with my body a full foot taller than hers, draped over her scapula.

Once in bed, Nivia props me up on a few pillows, and gingerly tucks in all the blankets. As I part my lips to issue some words of love, her hand comes so hard across my face it knocks the breath out of me. Disorientation floods my mind. I can't grasp where the slap has come from. Paranormal activity? Hallucination? I reason the fever is playing tricks on me, but then I see Nivia trembling. Her eyes meet mine, and I see they are solidly black. A cyclone of confusion grows between us and through the rotating blur of emotions I understand, abstractly, that my fainting spell has incited neuronal activity linking my current illness to Vivian's illness. The overlap of past and present caused the slap to fly out of Nivia involuntarily, so now we sit together on the bed with the anger, the love, and the fear whirring around us. I realize this whole time she hasn't been interfacing with me, but some shimmer of genetic information fluctuating over my face like a hologram. She only sees her daughter, who is sick and dying once more.

"Don't you ever do that again," she says to her through me, and then she leaves the room, shutting the door behind her so she can forget this ever happened.

CRISPR

In 1987, researchers at Osaka University working with *E. coli* bacteria discovered a genomic anomaly: clusters consisting of a short, specific DNA sequence followed by a segment of "spacer DNA" (i.e., noncoding DNA) were repeated throughout its code. These clusters occurred at "regularly spaced intervals," making them a chorus in the *E. coli*'s genomic ballad. However, unlike a typical refrain, these clusters did not enhance the ensuing melody. They did not code for any functions, essential or otherwise, or produce proteins, and thus presented as garbage, which flew in the face of scientific belief. It is widely held that patterns found within the natural world are indicative of purpose, and thus are not ornamental or accidental. Flummoxed by this seeming incongruity, the researchers spent the next several years trying to determine the nature of these clusters. Experiments were repeated, heads were bashed into walls, results remained elusive. The only concrete development was in the nomenclature department: the anomaly was given the name CRISPR, or "clustered regularly interspersed short palindromic repeats."

There are many moments within scientific history in which progress is botched by adherence to a certain viewpoint. The case of CRISPR is no exception, and ultimately it was a computer that exploded the situational context. During the years researchers toiled away in Osaka, computer technology dramatically evolved. This advent had many scientific applications, one of them being the ability to process genetic sequences at unprecedented rates. Large-scale genomic databases began popping up and, as a result, researchers were suddenly able to cross-reference DNA samples on a global scale with ease. In 2005, the mystery *E. coli* sequence was fed into such a database and was matched, astonishingly, to a virus. Effectively, the CRISPR researchers lacked the imagination to view the clusters beyond a bacterial context. Their hardened perspective crippled their own investigation.

This viral dimension added a new plot twist to CRISPR. The mystery cluster was identified as belonging to a bacteriophage, or a type of virus that feasts exclusively on *E. coli*. On both scientific and philosophical levels this was earth-shattering; for an organism to possess, within the intimate folds of its genome, DNA belonging to its archnemesis made absolutely no sense. The problem would require severe lateral thinking, and fortunately famed computational biologist Eugene Koonin was up to the task. Well known for his eccentricities, in addition to his work, Koonin managed to channel the *E. coli* sensibility into his own brain and surmise that the viral DNA was actually an integral component of *E. coli*'s immune system. This hypothesis turned out to be correct.

CRISPR works like this: in the highly unusual event that a bacterium survives a viral infection caused by a bacteriophage, its immune system sends out an enzyme, called Cas9, to cut up any remaining viral fragments. The enzyme then captures and deposits these fragments into the CRISPR slots of the bacteria's genome, where it becomes, in Koonin's words, "a mug shot." In the future, if the bacterium is infected with the same virus, its immune system will reference the shot and immediately deploy the exact defenses to crush the attack. Over time the bacterial immune system will create something akin to an album of mug shots, or "a most-wanted gallery" of villains. CRISPR has also been likened to a memory storage device, such as a hard drive or USB stick.

The profound excitement surrounding CRISPR is the adaptability of the mechanism. It has been recognized as a completely natural gene-editing technology that can be applied to any organism, including humans. The Cas9 enzyme can effectively be "programmed" to locate and cut out specific segments of DNA, thereby resulting in definitive physiological changes. For instance, CRISPR could be used to eliminate and replace errant genes in the human genome, like the ones that cause Huntington's or Lou Gehrig's disease. The power of CRISPR is literally awesome, but as with anything this powerful, there is also a dark side. If we can edit out disease, we can also edit out other features like hair color, height, and intelligence. The genome could be tailored to a set of preferences, not unlike a dating profile.

MIDLIFE CRISIS/UNEXPECTED VICTORY

In 2009 the internet turns forty, a milestone for something once billed as a "fad invention." Most major media outlets run stories about this, though none are particularly insightful beyond their tendency to regard the events of the last four decades just as a person might when reflecting on their life at this delicate juncture.

IT WAS A DARK AND STORMY NIGHT

At an empty bar in a hotel, I stash my dripping umbrella under a stool and order a manhattan. The night is gelatinous and black, full of rain and other things that make going out distinctly unappealing. The bartender, for lack of things to do, starts chatting with me. We exchange pleasantries, and eventually, through a protracted exchange, it comes out that he's a musician and I'm an artist, which is a fact I prefer to keep hidden because it pains me to answer the inevitable follow-up question—"What kind of art do you make?"— especially when I suspect the person's frame of reference is Monet, *The Da Vinci Code,* or Damien Hirst's shark.

"So, what kind of art do you make?" he asks while buffing a wineglass.

"I work with . . . words and pictures basically. My background is photography, but mostly I just try to convey moods through images, so sometimes that involves writing. Right now I'm starting a project about Los Angeles in the eighties. That's where I'm from, originally."

"You sound a lot like my sister. She's an artist too, getting her MA at Goldsmiths."

"Artistic genes must run in the family."

A drenched soul pushes through the revolving door and takes a place by the fire. The bartender goes to deal with him and I stare at the myriad bottles glowing like precious stones on the glass shelves. The metallic rustle of a cocktail shaker followed by ice tumbling in a glass hits like a familiar song; it's the kind of night when sensorial information is magnified and plays on one's heartstrings, so by the time the bartender comes back I feel flush enough to pose the dreaded question, "What kind of art does your sister make?"

He's not really clear, "to be honest," on what it is she does, he just knows it involves an inordinate amount of time in the library. She does however produce a monthly zine called *The Hawl*, which consists of photocopied imagery and essays on gender politics. She also "performs" slideshow presentations, narrating fictions over slides she's bought at flea markets.

"I'm not sure what you'd call that mixture," he says.

"No one is," I say.

"She'd like your project though, I think. Going back in time into another place, a legendary one."

"Is she any good at the practical version of that sort of thing? Research? Digging up old documents?"

"She has friends who are better at it than she is."

"Anyone who might be looking for some side work?"

"Paid?"

"Absolutely."

"Let me find out."

He goes over to his phone plugged in discreetly by the rum shelf, sends out a message, and then we wait. The second coming of Christ seems more likely to happen in the next thirty minutes than any leads from this interaction.

More customers, soggy with the residue of the week, perch at the opposite end of the bar. I fold my cocktail napkin into different shapes, stab the orange peel in my drink with the stirrer. From the corner of my eye, I see a series of boxes glow across the bartender's phone. A deep bellow of thunder, followed by some lightning, kills the murmur of the room. A hush falls. The thunder crashes again, and an older gentleman raises his glass to the ceiling. Laughter and motion resume.

The bartender takes this opportunity to check his phone. He scribbles something down on the back of a coaster, slides it over to me across the mahogany bar, and says, "Here's the info for some friend of a friend of Georgia's." I take a look. There's an 818 number followed by the name Katherine.

"Is this girl in California? The Valley?"

"No idea. Hey, are you okay?"

I feel like Christ just came in through the door.

PARTING

Parting contracts the distance between people while simultaneously splitting them apart.

DOCTORS AND DETECTIVES

Conceptualizing medicine, and by extension the body, from militaristic or mechanistic standpoints has unintended consequences for our understanding. Inevitably, diagnostic facts are twisted away from their neutral reality and into other territories that support the employed metaphor. A possible resolution to this issue would be the implementation of less charged and more nuanced frameworks to the disease/health paradigm. For example, the Medicine-as-a-Detective-Story proposition offers a noninvasive yet natural parallel to the diagnostic process. Illness, after all, unfolds in time and requires narrative to capture it. Patients relay their symptoms in the form of a chronological story to a doctor who then, like a detective, examines the account. Though the doctor's means of investigation differ from the detective's, utilizing tests, scans, and cultures to gather evidence, both professionals ultimately seek to solve their cases through hard facts, and even the shared use of the term "case" implies an organic, philosophical correspondence between the fields.

This is perhaps not accidental. Resonance between these figures can be traced to the emergence of a diagnostic practice popularized during the nineteenth century. The practice, known as clinical reasoning, is a system of deductive analysis wherein the totality of the doctor's expertise and experience as a human being works as a siphon to home in on a diagnosis. It requires several capacities such as the "ability to integrate and apply different types of knowledge . . . weigh evidence, critically think about arguments and to reflect upon the process used to arrive at a diagnosis."

The X factor of clinical reasoning is, in fact, the mind of the doctor and its unique cocktail of intuition and knowledge:

It looks easy on television, but the capacity to perceive and assign correct values to internal discrepancies requires a command of the entire diagnostic scenario. This talent needs a blend of observational capacity, logical reasoning, culture, and abductive imagination.

Clinical reasoning begins with an interview wherein the patient's current symptoms, current lifestyle, and past medical history are documented. The doctor then synthesizes these elements to create a diagnostic theory, while also keeping an eye toward what's not there:

> If one investigative quality marks out the mature clinician it is the ability to spot possible inconsistencies among the clinical, instrumental, and laboratory examinations, considering not only what is present but also what is missing. This requires skills in observation and "deduction," handling of knowledge, pattern recognition, and the astuteness that comes from years of experience.

Through tests the diagnostic theory is refined, and a treatment plan is put into play. Changes in the patient's health data will further solidify or crumble the correctness of the theory.

Prior to the mid-1800s, physicians performed these tasks haphazardly. Their organization into a dynamic practice consequently transformed the medical field. An early proponent of this new practice was Dr. Joseph Bell, a highly decorated Scottish surgeon. Bell first made a name for himself at the tender age of twenty-nine by penning the authoritative volume *A Manual of the Operations of Surgery*. Later he became the president of the Royal College of Surgeons of Edinburgh, where he championed women's rights in medical education, and held the distinction of being Queen Victoria's on-call physician. His early adoption of clinical reasoning thus imbued it with an attractive air, which in turn promoted it, but beyond this and his other achievements, Bell was renowned for one other talent: his near-supernatural powers of observation. Allegedly he could discern a patient's profession, most recent whereabouts, and neighborhood of residence simply by scanning their appearance. He performed this feat on many a social occasion, but beyond being a party trick, he stressed observation as part of medical education:

In teaching the treatment of disease and accident, all careful teachers have first to show the student how to recognise accurately the case. The recognition depends in great measure on the accurate and rapid appreciation of *small* points in which the diseased differs from the healthy state. In fact, the student must be taught to observe. To interest him in this kind of work we teachers find it useful to show the student how much a trained use of the observation can discover in ordinary matters such as the previous history, nationality, and occupation of a patient.

In 1877, one of Bell's students became his personal clerk: Arthur Conan Doyle, later Sir Arthur Conan Doyle, or the creator of the world's greatest detective: Sherlock Holmes.

TRAVEL BAN

In 2010, President Barack Obama lifts the HIV Travel and Immigration Ban, which was enacted in 1987 and formalized by Congress in 1993. The ban prohibited people living with HIV/AIDS from immigrating or traveling to the US. In accordance with this, the Department of Health and Human Services listed HIV as a "communicable disease of public health significance" alongside leprosy, tuberculosis, and other highly infectious diseases caused by airborne contagion or casual contact. At the time, it was well documented that HIV was not transmissible via these mechanisms, making the ban entirely prejudicial. In 1989, the brutality of the legislation crystalized when Dutch educator Hans Paul Verhoef, traveling en route to San Francisco as a delegate for two health conferences, was detained in jail for six days after confirming his HIV-positive status at passport control. In a show of solidarity with Verhoef and other patients, all international AIDS conferences boycotted US soil from 1990 onward. The end of the ban is meant to mend this rift in the global HIV/AIDS community and herald a new age of information exchange.

ENZYME

I am fixated on the enzyme hacking up fragments of viral code and inserting them into the genome—or rather, I'm caught in the metaphor of it, of the code becoming a picture and then existing as part of the organism. A bell goes off in my mind; an entity partially composed of images, of ones scavenged from the outside, seems . . . familiar. I think I've been trying to rewrite myself in a similar way. I think I've been trying to edit my own code with scenes nicked from movies and television shows over the years. They fill in the empty spaces of my lineage, creating albums of coherent pasts and visions of possible futures.

DAD FRAGMENTS

I have a string of images connected to David that I am mostly sure have been lifted from photographs, yet they constitute the majority of my remembrances of him. In this string, David is only ever semi-visible. He either looms as a dense shadow, or appears pixelated like an anonymized figure on reality TV. This is, of course, a trick of memory, and sometimes he is even broken down into segments of an elbow or a nose that appear in tantalizingly sharp focus while the rest of him fades. Inconsequential details blossom and are magnified within the frame to compensate for the loss of their central character, and this disproportion magnetically draws my attention. I fixate on the most mundane objects as if they contain a lifetime of love within them.

Here is the string:

- The gray rubber eyepiece of a camcorder pressed against an oily eye socket with tiny red veins running away from it
- A hand lifted dramatically over a Smith Corona typewriter
- Another hand unfolding the neck joints of a desk lamp so large and unwieldy it resembles an exotic bird
- Gangly knees and calves pedaling a razor-thin bicycle
- A raised band of cream cable-knit flowing down the shoulder of a sweater

Beyond this, there is only the dim and pervasive awareness that my presence was a near-constant irritation to him.

LESS ABOUT INTERPRETATION

"Cognition is an intellectual activity which depends on the rational faculties. Seeing, witnessing, over-looking, watching, are all—though they assist in the cognitive process (by prompting intuition or leading to perception)—more instinctive, visceral activities than reasoning, less easy to control or direct. While what a detective sees is closely linked to what he knows, interpretation is less the concern in private eye movies than spectacle."

—*The Private Eye:*
Detectives in the Movies
by Bran Nicol

215

WHEN A PERSON DIES

When a person is born, whatever will kill them is already inside them, and what they think of the world will grow over it like a skin.

When a person dies, their life is read in reverse in particles that ricochet in the minds of their friends, with the last encounter gleaming like a shard of glass in the sand.

AIRPORT ARRIVAL

On the curb of the arrivals section of LAX, I stand in a pool of solid shadow. Chemical fumes of gasoline and tar pluck at my nostrils while the "loading and unloading of passengers" announcement played on a loop distorts all other auditory signals. Jet lag fills my head with sand. I catch thoughts one at a time, as if with tweezers, and place them on a line in the hope an idea will appear. After twenty minutes, all I've gathered is: how does a person fly over five thousand miles without a plan of what to do upon arrival?

Absentmindedly, I wander onto a shuttle bus and sit in the back. I have a dim notion that it will deposit me at a Hertz or an Enterprise, but by the time I've committed to this reality I realize I'm on a different type of shuttle and get ejected into a parking lot miles away from the terminals. No one else gets off with me. In fact, there is no one else to disembark except the driver, who screeches away as soon as I'm out the door. The merciless 2 P.M. sun is milky white and drips over the barren expanse of concrete. I walk across the lot to something vaguely resembling a tree. Surprisingly it provides a morsel of shade despite its near-total lack of branches.

Other than some weeds, it is the only hint of nature as far as the eye can see. A seagull touches down on a lamppost and glares at me. Then another joins it, and glares at me too.

I perch on my suitcase when my brain finally decides to chime in: you got into this situation because you are a *fucking moron*. I put on my sunglasses because instead of being cold and clinical right now, I am going to cry. In this exact moment, in a parallel universe, I am riding in a Subaru station wagon alongside my mother doing the breakdown of my flight, or I'm with my best friend in her beat-up Jeep Cherokee listening to her latest work drama, or I'm on the curb when my boyfriend rolls up in a vintage Porsche with a bouquet of roses . . . I take a deep breath and blow all those other lives away.

I figure I'll sit here and cry until the shuttle returns. Unfortunately, this could be at any time. In ten minutes, an hour, every other hour. It's free transport in LA after all. I crumple then, on my knockoff Away carry-on, but just as I give in to total despair the sound of a motor draws my attention. A black Chevy Impala turns in to the lot. It zooms toward me, and then abruptly stops. The driver lowers the passenger window and shouts, "Are you my two o'clock?" over a plane taking off.

"Nope."

"You're not the Wassermans?"

"No, I, ah, I'm just one person."

"But you're a Wasserman?"

"No. Sorry. I was trying to make a joke."

"So you don't have a reservation with Charlie Parker's Rent 'n Fly?"

"You're a rental agency?"

"A small one. Among other things."

For a minute we stop talking and let the sounds of jet engines fill in whatever it is that is happening.

"What are you doing here?" she says.

I open my mouth to say something and then close it again.

"You look like you could use a lift," she says, moving her aviators to her forehead with a fingertip.

I get off my suitcase and roll with it to the car window to continue the conversation. "I got the wrong shuttle. I was trying to get to Hertz or National. Now I'm stranded."

"Well, we got cars."

And before I know it, I'm in the passenger seat hurtling down Century Boulevard toward who knows what.

COMMUNICATING VIA IMAGES

In 2010, a free photo-sharing app for iPhone is launched. Capitalizing on the ubiquity of the Apple device, Instagram allows seamless integration between taking photos and sharing them on a social media platform. Once uploaded to the app, photos are sized in a retro, 1:1 square format. They can then be manipulated with a variety of filters and editing tools. Posts are made visible to users' followers in a feed, which, over time, develops into a near-infinite scroll of eye candy. Instagram differs from other photo-sharing apps in a particularly potent way. Rather than focus on static image preservation, the app is built around the concept of "communicating via images." This insight, into what is essentially a new language, is the key to Instagram's popularity. In the first year of its existence, it amasses ten million users, and as the app grows to include Android users it also incorporates video, messaging, shopping, live feeds, reels, and stories into its features. However, these additions shift its purpose. Instagram becomes a tool to "build influence" rather than a quick means to share (casual) images of one's life.

AIDS DISKETTE

The Joseph L. Popp, Jr. Butterfly Conservatory sits on State Route 7 in New York. On Google Street View this is a two-lane road bordered by fields and pine trees. An unceremonious gravel turnoff leads to the entrance of the conservatory, which is open all year long. Prime butterfly viewing season occurs in mid-to-late summer, when both heat and daylight stretch as far as they can go. The other main attraction is a menagerie of reptiles and tropical plants housed in a three-thousand-square-foot indoor garden, which you can enter for around ten dollars, or less if you're a student or over sixty-five.

The Conservatory was founded by its namesake and his daughter sometime after 1990. Prior to this, Dr. Popp, an evolutionary biologist, was embroiled in the world's premier cyber-terror scandal. The crime involved encrypting data through ransomware distributed on floppy disks. In the UK, Popp was charged with ten counts of blackmail but ultimately walked free. The case was dismissed as Popp was declared "unfit to stand trial." To this day, this "diagnosis" as well as the motivation for his actions remain questionable. The most oft-played scenario chalks it up to an overlooked job promotion: Popp was a part-time AIDS researcher for the World Health Organization. He applied for a full-time position but was rejected. A few months later, twenty thousand medical professionals in ninety different countries had their digitized lives seized and dissolved.

The victims of the scheme, all affiliated with the WHO or the 1988 International AIDS Conference, received a diskette in the mail. Issued by the PC Cyborg Corporation, it was innocuously labeled AIDS INFORMATION INTRODUCTORY DISKETTE but contained something decidedly not innocuous, a "Trojan horse" virus. As its name suggests, this species of virus sits beneath a fully operational façade program and quietly downloads in the background. In this case, the façade program behaved as a risk calculator, mathematically determining a patient's risk of contracting HIV based on answers to a questionnaire. For eighty-nine reboots, users interfaced normally with their machines, but on the ninetieth, the Trojan virus sprang to life, encrypting the user's files. Because of the targeted demographic, the majority of these files consisted of HIV/AIDS data assembled through years of painstaking clinical efforts, meaning the world was now cut off from potentially lifesaving information. There was, however, one solution: a payment of a $189 "software licensing fee" could be mailed to a PO box in Panama. Once processed, a decryption key would be dispatched to the victim, also through the mail.

Extortion exercised through computer technology was revolutionary. No one knew how to react. Some people obediently paid the ransom, others voluntarily destroyed their hard drives, erasing years of research. Law enforcement from Interpol to the FBI proceeded to scour the planet for a mustache-stroking technological mastermind, or a genius hacker with a spiked orange mohawk. Not a single professional imagined the architect of the diskette to be a disgruntled biologist who may or may not have purposefully outed himself as the villain: on his way home to Ohio from an AIDS seminar in Nairobi, Popp wrote on a passenger's suitcase

DR. POPP HAS BEEN POISONED. During his layover at Schiphol airport authorities pulled him aside to question him about this curious graffiti. At the commencement of the interview Popp's luggage was searched and dozens of labels for the now-infamous PC Cyborg Corp. spilled out of his bags. The FBI was notified and upon his arrival in the US, Popp was immediately extradited to the UK. At this point, his unusual behavior became even more pronounced. According to *The Atlantic*, Popp "wore condoms on his nose and curlers in his beard to protect from radiation" during pretrial motions. The judge, either not wanting to engage with Popp's mental state or the monumental task of establishing precedents in a completely new realm of the law, declared a mistrial. The ransomware became known as the AIDS Trojan.

Popp died in 2007. There is no reference to his cause of death or more than a line about his daughter anywhere on the internet, at least that I can find.

EQUIVALENTS

Photographer Alfred Stieglitz began a series of images in 1922 that he would eventually title *Equivalents*. The images were taken of the sky above his home and were printed on silver gelatin. At the Tate Modern four of them are on display and from across the room they cut a sharp metallic horizon line over the white wall of the gallery. Each photograph looks like a ghost in various states of diffusion printed on a mirror. In one, clouds are pulled thin in a sheet, in another they streak across the frame in a dense mass, as if being chased. The blurs and textures of their figures are evasive and the monochromatic scale removes the context of day or night. At a passing glance these photographs would appear only as graphic abstractions, and in a sense, they are; in Stieglitz's mind these are not photos of the sky, but a reflection of an interior state. The cloud formations correspond to personal feelings. "Shapes, as such, mean nothing to me, unless I happen to be feeling something within, of which an equivalent appears, in outer form."

I get as close as possible to one of the prints until my field of vision is overwhelmed with black. The rest of the frame only contains jagged wisps of white as if a claw shredded a cumulus. If you didn't know this was a picture of the sky, you wouldn't be able to see it. It would rest in the mind as a series of lines and shadows, or perhaps smoke. You might see the echo of violence, or something in the process of dissolving, but nothing specific you could name.

On the opposite wall is a quote: "What is of greatest importance is to hold a moment, to record something so completely that those who see it will relive an equivalent of what has been expressed."

To hold. There it is again.

THE END OF THE UNIVERSE

I drag myself into the living room, my heavy duvet a tidal wave behind me. On the couch I curl up inside it like a hermit crab. I flick on the TV and channel surf with the smallest possible sliver of my index finger. It's 3:30 A.M. and a chill hangs in the air. Onscreen *Poirot, EastEnders,* infomercials for weight-loss products, reruns of the *Real Housewives of Whatever the Fuck,* and ads for payday loans, online casinos, and dating websites for "mature love seekers" play out. I mindlessly click until I land on glowing balls of gas streaking across a sky. A trail of white dotted lines appears behind them, marking out a geometric trajectory in a swath of darkness. It's an alluring computer animation of a space event. The colors are unfamiliar to the eye, and the action of the comets, or perhaps meteorites, takes place in a heavy silence that erases the lingering chatter of the previous images. The next shot is of a giant antenna dish blossoming out of sand like an orchid. The info caption says this is a BBC production called *The Beginning and the End of the Universe,* so I keep on clicking. My anxiety level for the state of the world is already at a fever pitch, and considering the fate of the entire universe on top of that seems like not a good choice. I resume scanning garbage, and after a brief foray into an episode of *The Kardashians,* where Kim performs her first (and let's face it, probably last) keg stand, I gravitate back to the BBC show.

A few minutes in, a strange solace melts through my chest. My index finger retracts into my palm, and respiration becomes less constricted. The end of the universe is perhaps the only cataclysmic event humans can't be responsible for. Try as we might, we actually cannot destroy everything. There are elements so vast and mysterious in their workings they exist far beyond our scope of interference, and for some reason, this knowledge quiets my heart.

The host, Professor Jim Al-Khalili, is a tall, jovial man elegantly dressed in slacks and a Barbour jacket. His height seems in danger of bursting out of frame, which speaks to his presence as much as it does his physique. He is so acutely comfortable on camera I wonder whether he's missed his calling as an actor. Professor Jim has that certain je ne sais quoi that radiates straight through the lens. The content he shares makes him visibly effervescent, and this bubbling excitement seems to incite a constant change of scenery. His lectures pop across a tapas restaurant in northern Spain, a candlelit tunnel, the chalk cliffs of an English coastline, and the interior of a red Fiat sedan, all somewhat unusual locations for an educational program.

In each setting he deploys props and other visual aids to enhance his arguments. Black-and-white photographs of scientists are pulled out of jacket pockets and held up during monologues. A handful of marbles, produced from yet another jacket pocket, is at one point dropped into a dish and swirled around to mimic the movement of galaxies. In another scene, the professor creates a chart representing the life cycle of a star with rocks and boulders gathered in a forest but: *why is he in a forest?* The more I watch the less I can tell if my state of mind is causing this crackle in reality, or if the show itself is bordering on the surreal, but it continues to glide by with glossy images so easy on the eyes it feels like drinking. I become so enthralled with the pictures I lose complete track of the physics. I think only of what a nice life it must be to work as a cinematographer for a BBC science show, to do something creative yet purposeful, with a definitive job title, that could make your parents proud. . . . A shift in light causes the reverie to disintegrate, and all the particles of my room, books, posters, loose socks, lock into sharp focus.

On the program, Prof Jim sits in the sterile control room of a lab with many buttons and huge windows. He describes an event from 1973 in which the Jodrell Bank observatory conducted a survey of quasars using the Lovell Telescope, then the largest radio telescope in the world. Quasars, or quasi-stellar objects, are hyperluminous phenomena consisting of supermassive black holes and accretion disks. They are rare and notoriously difficult to find. Hunting them amounts to aiming a telescope at a quadrant of space and scanning through it for particular radio signatures. This process is not dissimilar to searching for a needle in a haystack, even with the help of the magnificent Lovell, so it came as a massive shock when not one but *two* quasars appeared in stunningly close proximity to each other. On a gut level the researchers knew this had to be a mistake and assumed they had inadvertently identified the same quasar twice. However, the data proved otherwise: the frequencies of each quasar showed distinct variance, suggesting they were indeed separate entities. Confounded, the researchers took a radical approach and reconsidered the visual relationship of the two quasars. It could be, they reasoned, that the second quasar was actually a reflection of the first. For this to be true, gravity would have to form a "lens" in front of the real quasar; gravitational lensing occurs when a massive object, such as a galaxy, is stationed between a light source and an observer. The intense gravity of the massive object is such that it pulls any light radiating behind it off its natural trajectory, resulting in an optical distortion. Often the effect is that of a bright halo, or lens, around the massive object, but a reflection is equally plausible. While this seemed like a solid hypothesis, there was just one problem: there was no massive object in the vicinity to cause the lensing. The space around the quasars was empty.

There was only one possible explanation for this: the mystery object had to be dark matter. Considered theoretical until this moment, dark matter was something of a placeholder concept created to satisfy mathematical concerns about the universe. Basically, "unseen," or dark, matter must be present to prevent galaxies from flying apart. The numbers infer its existence, but it has no properties that we can optically—or otherwise—observe. In fact, it can only be perceived through its disruptions of gravity, meaning that for all intents and purposes, it is invisible. In 1973, the researchers at Jodrell Bank observatory believed a wedge of dark matter bent gravity in such a way as to generate a virtual quasar. This was an observable phenomenon that, through reverse engineering, revealed the presence of a previously undetectable type of matter.

I switch off the TV and stay sitting in the dark for a long time. I don't want to know how this all connects to the end of the universe. I just want to be still and think about all the things right in front of my face that I cannot see, but can feel, revolving, as the morning very gently seeps in under the blinds.

INSTRUMENTAL RESOURCES

The long-established congressional ban on the transplantation of HIV-infected organs is brought to public debate in 2011. Many healthcare professionals advocate for its removal, as allowing access to HIV-infected organs would save the lives of HIV-positive patients, a population historically denied transplantation. Research published in *The New England Journal of Medicine* is used to support this position. A recent study of kidney transplants found the survival rates of HIV-positive patients were close to that of older, HIV-negative patients, contradicting the long-held belief that HIV-positive patients were too immunosuppressed to benefit from organ donation.

At the same time, in other parts of the world, Twitter and Facebook are cited as instrumental resources in orchestrating the protests of the Arab Spring.

NOTES ON OBSERVATION

The action of observation requires a subject and an object. It is a Person and a Thing configuration, except sometimes that Thing might be another person, and the Person sometimes might be an AI. Categories of identity become indeterminate here. They bleed into each other to form a circuit, but the point really is: observation is a relationship.

GATES CLOSING

I want to say more about them, my parents, but each time I withdraw into memory, I feel metal gates closing in on me. My mind grows dim; light empties out from the images inside it. Details are erased. Faces are erased. Emotions turn cloudlike, vaporous, and yet some metadata is retained, like the sensation of love.

INTERNET STORY

They are at a nightclub and 2004 is hanging on by a thread. The nightclub is in Philadelphia with a lot of nostalgic black light and neon scattered along its crusty walls. Patrons are decked out in pleather, torn denim, and sweat. There are fishnet stockings, Vans, and small round badges pinned onto messenger bags. "Yeah!" by Usher blares through the speakers. Maybe there is even a disco ball twirling in a spotlight. The two approach opposite ends of the bar from opposite sides of the dance floor at approximately the same moment. He orders a vodka soda, she orders a Yuengling for three dollars, then the crowd between them disperses, clinking bottles and ironically fist pumping the air. The guy swirls his drink, stabs the lime wedge at the bottom of his glass with his straw, and casually attempts to unglue his arm from the bar top. While doing so, he looks down and sees the girl, sipping her beer, and velcroing her wallet back together. He knows her from somewhere. Her rounded posture and inked-up arms are detonating bells in his mind. As he studies the topsails and flags of the galleon on her biceps the girl turns to look at him. Her eyebrows temporarily furrow, then she walks up to him.

"Hey."

"Hey?"

"I know you," she says, "from the internet."

GETTING THE CAR

In the early nineties, Century Boulevard, at least from a child's perspective, felt like an epic city in its own right, with office buildings sharp and narrow as blades reflecting the noonday sun. It was the name partially that evoked this vision, as if the promise of a period of years, i.e., The Future, could be embedded on a stretch of concrete extending directly from the airport. At the time, Century was home to several "state-of-the-art" developments that advertised the most "advanced facilities" money could buy, and for a brief moment, familiar corporations came to inhabit them. Some even set up international headquarters, but little by little the grime appeared. The future moved elsewhere, and strange, two-bit enterprises replaced it, import-export dealers, lunchtime salad bars, one-hour passport photo shops, nail salons, and travel agencies with faded posters of safaris lining their windows.

The office for Charlie Parker's Rent 'n Fly is one of these businesses. Located on the ground floor of a massive tower block, it takes up an entire corner suite that looks like it was gutted yesterday during an emergency. The frenzy of whatever happened before, of ripped-out ethernet cords and smoking, shredded documents, lingers in the air, still nervously strumming its particles.

There are nail holes at uniform levels across two walls, and leftover cables piled over desks arranged in pod formations. The carpet in one corner carries a large rectangular indentation suggesting the ghost of a Xerox machine. A reception area at the front of the office remains nearly intact, except a passageway has been sloppily sawed into its waist-high countertop. Sheila, the lady who rescued me from the parking lot, sashays through it. "Hey, Charlie, I think the Wassermans died," she calls out before disappearing into the back. For a brief second, I hear a few notes of a clarinet, but that seems unreasonable. Clearly, I'm more exhausted than I thought, hearing music in the low hum of the ventilation system.

I maneuver myself to the one available chair and sit in it. Next to me is an artificial rubber tree whose leaves have acquired about ten years' worth of dust. A small table holds a stack of *Ebony* magazines from 2009. I casually flip through one and read an article about "Mother, Rocker, Actor, Wife" Jada Pinkett Smith. I flip through the whole issue, roll it into a tube, and look through it.

On the wall arranged in a diagonal line are four black-and-white headshots. One of them I recognize as a younger version of Sheila with a Princess Diana haircut and velveteen V-neck. Above her is an Asian guy, lanky as a straw and outfitted in a bow tie. He looks cheeky and stoic in equal measures. Next up is a man whom I nickname Mr. Saturday Night on account of his grin and cigar, and the final image of the line is of a petite Black woman flirtatiously glancing over her shoulder, a diamond drop earring framing her face. My eyes pull themselves up and down the staircase of these shots and then to a nearby print for a jazz festival, which covers a door. The print is designed in the constructivist vein, with geometric slices of red and black interrupting photographic imagery of brass instruments. As I start to read the text the door swings open and a person tumbles out. It's an older version of the Asian guy in the headshot. I drop my magazine telescope, tossing it back on the table nonchalantly like I've done nothing weird.

"Sorry to keep you waiting," he says, rushing across the room, arm stiffly extended in front of him. "I'm Charlie."

We meet at the counter and our hands click into place. "Heather."

"Stop flirting with her, Charlie. This girl needs a car to get on with her life," Sheila calls out from some nonvisible location.

"Oh, you're one to talk. I bet you chatted her up the entire way over here. Besides, all I've done so far is give her a handshake."

Outside, the sun drops into a crack between two buildings, which funnel its rays directly through the rental agency. They illuminate the central channel of the office space, as well as Charlie, who seems to have walked right off the wall and into my life. The manner he projects in his headshot is now happening before me, in three dimensions.

Sheila emerges with two coffee cups.

"Thanks," says Charlie.

"It's not for you, it's for her. She's like on an eight-hour time difference and she's drooping."

I take the coffee and nod.

"Where are you joining us from?" Charlie asks.

"London."

He takes out an iPad and starts working out the rental details. I give him my driver's license and credit card and request their cheapest/most generic car model, which somehow turns out to be a problem. Their fleet is composed solely of "specialty" cars, the least offensive of which is a lilac Mini Cooper with racing decals. I sigh, sign the screen, and sit back down by the rubber tree.

"What brings you to LA?" asks Charlie.

"I'm here to meet a private detective."

"Oh, nice," he says, without so much as a glance up from his iPad.

The silence following his remark is broken by an ungodly blast from a trombone.

"Holy fuck!" inadvertently bursts from my mouth.

"Oh, that's just the boys."

"The boys?"

"Yeah, they're on tonight. You should stick around if you can stay awake—"

"On *where?*"

"Downstairs."

"Downstairs?"

"Yes."

"It's a nightclub?"

He nods.

"You're joking."

"You just heard the trombone."

"I'm sorry, people actually come here for live music?"

"There's a basement that is theoretically only accessible through this office, but you can get to it through the subterranean parking garage where we keep the rentals."

I can only imagine that the agreement with building management, if there even is one, is unconventional at best.

"My friends and I"—he juts his chin toward the headshots—"just wanted a place to rehearse and we came across this place in a series of . . . events. We used to play all around town, for years, but then Maxine got sick and things changed after she went . . . We didn't really like performing without her, but we missed the show atmosphere, and, well, downstairs turned into The Nest."

A telephone rings, or rather, a burner phone shivers on an empty desk. Charlie grabs it. "This is Parker's Rent 'n Fly . . . Oh, Mrs. Wasserman! My deepest apologies—"

Eventually Sheila shows up with the rental keys, but I ask her if I can see The Nest before I take off. She opens the door with the jazz poster and leads me down a narrow stairwell that smells of chlorine. At the bottom is another door with the silver silhouette of a bird painted underneath a peephole. She cracks it open, and I slip inside a very skinny room with a leather banquette on one side and a zinc bar top on the other. The banquette and the bar both dead-end at a stage with a bloodred curtain behind it. The stage is impossibly small, raised only about a foot off the ground, and yet a quartet—with their instruments—looks comfortably arranged. They are hyper-focused, discussing a controversial tempo change, and hardly notice Sheila and me. Besides, the place is so dim I'm sure we don't look like much beyond shadows. I try to catch our reflections in the antique mirror above the bar, which doesn't so much stretch the space as fold into it an extreme dimension of darkness. Flecked with a million gold veins, it's beautiful and oh, so Parisian. The liquor shelves are also mirrored and hold fake tea lights programmed to flicker. I take a last look around and notice a framed cookie fortune above the host's stand. "May you live in interesting times."

PrEP

In 2012, the FDA approves the antiretroviral drug Truvada for use as a pre-exposure prophylaxis (PrEP) for individuals at risk of contracting HIV. Taken as a once-a-day prescription, Truvada reduces the risk of HIV infection through sex by 99 percent and intravenous drug use by 74 percent.

BLOOD

I didn't have much in me. I spent it all thinking about blood and what's in it that makes us prioritize certain people over others. Blood, after all, is the source and also price of every conflict, but it is only code. It shows lineage but it doesn't show relation. Blood is information without the story. I drove around and thought about this because resonance on the genetic level doesn't always translate into responsibility, love, or respect, which makes me believe that family bonds are just as invented as all our other bonds. We make such a dramatic fuss over blood ties and yet people are just people. It's all artifice. The truth is, you're dead lucky if your mother actually loves you as a *person,* and not just because you came out of her body.

MAP

I clear out the storage shed in the backyard. The shed holds all the pieces of a life that cannot be boxed up and stored in a hallway closet, like a full-size artificial fruit tree, a collapsible card table, a bolt of polyester fabric, and an epic tangle of Christmas lights. Behind all these relics, against the wall, is a map of the world. It is glued to a sheet of cardboard, and to reach it I must chisel out a path, excavating a three-piece luggage set and a television monitor from the "memento" accretion in the process. I set these items in the sun to decompress, the sharp imprints of my hands caught in their skins of dust. The map, now freed, slides through the door, and I take it inside for further inspection.

In the kitchen, Nivia washes dishes with the radio on. She has it tuned to a Latin jazz station, and she shifts her weight from one foot to the other in a simple cha-cha-cha as she rinses. I put the map on the dining room table and see immediately it is beyond saving. Water damage has caused the paper to bubble away from the cardboard, imbuing it with novel topographical features, and an aroma of mildew emanates from the Atlantic Ocean. My eyes glide across speckles of fungal colonies to continents. The shades of individual countries prick at something lost in my memory. Lavender, mint green, pale orange, and yellow blend into a nostalgia gray; these faded renditions of space are no longer connected to time.

"What did you find, darling?" Nivia calls from the kitchen.

I hear the faucet shut off and then she is across from me, holding the barest edge of the map in her fingers. She grazes the paper gingerly and as she moves, the remaining adhesive gives way. I then notice an odd thing: a thick red marker line curling its way through every landmass. I look up at her face and somehow catch her not as she is, but how she must have been as a young woman. It is just a brief shiver of images colliding in my mind, but it leaves a trace. Even though her hands are now all skin and swollen joints, the echo of how they once moved across surfaces and through the air is superimposed over them.

"You found my map," she says.

One night, alone, after her second marriage imploded, Nivia took the folded-up map off the shelf. She looked at it and thought of all the places she had never been, then picked up a permanent marker and drew a path through each and every country, linking them together in a single red stroke. She would drive this line across the world, on her own, and it would be glorious.

"This was my own little secret. I never told this to anyone, except you."

LIFE GOALS?

1. For a life to assemble itself into a picture once seen in an app and then to have that new reality photographed, turned into a new image, and put back onto the same app, what is the name for this contemporary condition?

Or,

2. How would it feel to live a magazine life? To become an image of beauty and power in three-dimensional space? To exist in time as a full-bleed spread? Would you feel satisfied then?

ANTIVAXXER

The Persistence of Chaos is an artwork consisting of a 10.2-inch Samsung NC10 laptop and six of the most devastating pieces of malware in existence: BlackEnergy, Sobig, Dark Tequila, MyDoom, WannaCry, and ILOVEYOU. It was auctioned during a livestream in 2019 and sold for $1.35 million. The artist, Guo O Dong, was commissioned by Deep Instinct, a cybersecurity firm, to produce the work, which is meant to embody the seeming "abstract threats posed by the digital world." In an interview with artnet.com, Dong explains, "The piece emphasizes that internet and IRL are the same place. Placing these pieces of malware—which we ordinarily think of as remote processes happening somewhere on [a] network, but surely not to us—into this one crappy old laptop concretizes them." The title, a nod to Dalí's *The Persistence of Memory,* invokes the decay of the melting clocks, but more so, acknowledges the inevitability of chaos as a force; the combined toll of global economic fallout caused by the selected malware is upward of $95 billion.

For security purposes, the laptop was isolated and air-gapped to prevent any unwanted transmissions. The terms of sale for the auction read:

> The sale of malware for operational purposes is illegal in the United States. As a buyer you recognize that this work represents a potential security hazard. By submitting a bid you agree and acknowledge that you're purchasing this work as a piece of art or for academic reasons, and have no intention of disseminating any malware. Upon the conclusion of this auction and before the artwork is shipped, the computer's internet capabilities and available ports will be functionally disabled.

The project cost ten thousand dollars to fabricate and was originally titled *Antivaxxer.*

FLIGHT MH17

On July 17, 2014, six AIDS researchers and activists are killed on Malaysia Airlines flight MH17. The group traveling to the twentieth International AIDS Conference in Melbourne, Australia, was "hit by a surface-to-air missile supplied to pro-Russian rebels in eastern Ukraine." Speaking to *Time* magazine, Professor Brian Owler, president of the Australian Medical Association, stated, "The amount of knowledge that these people who died on the plane were carrying with them and the experiences they had developed will have a devastating impact on HIV research."

P.I. INTRO

I drive past the address she gave me, so I park on a side street and walk back to the main drag. For about a full minute everything seems promising. The address is either attached to a tiny, retro-looking architectural firm, or a dark twisty bar with a tiki-goth vibe. Either spot seems ideal for meeting the P.I. One screams hip-ster professionalism, the other cinematic mystery.

I am intrigued, to say the least. Through texting with her I've learned she's tracked down a colleague's birth mother and located someone else's uncle who went AWOL after a divorce. Google re-sults also show she has a "vibrant" art practice dealing with found objects. I've been vague with her in terms of my needs, preferring to relay it all face-to-face. I did give a passing mention to wanting re-search on some deceased LA citizens, and her response was "Cool," followed by an emoji face wearing sunglasses. I assumed at the time she meant this ironically or was perhaps in a whimsical mood, but now I'm not sure, as the address turns out to belong to a bubble tea parlor. I've flown halfway across the world to get boba in K-Town.

I walk in and Céline Dion is singing "Because You Loved Me." Seated at a lime-green table right next to the window is Katherine. She looks about six or seven years older than me, with a sharp face forged from many angles. Thick, black, rectangular frames add to this Cubist aesthetic, but her hair is all over the place. At one point it was probably in a bun held together by a pencil, as there is a pencil loosely hanging in her wild mane. She looks up from her reading material and sees me. "Heather!"

She stands up and goes in for a hug, but she's so tiny I have to sort of drape my body over hers to approximate the gesture.

"Thanks so much for meeting me here. They have free superfast Wi-Fi and my Airbnb is just around the corner."

"Oh, so you don't have an office? A shared workspace or studio—"

"God no. I travel, like, all the time, and don't want to be weighed down by contracts and leases—hey, do you want something? Let me get you something." And then she leaves to order.

I have purposefully avoided boba tea for my entire life. It's a texture thing.

Her laptop is open on the table. I make an elaborate yet nonchalant bend of my body to glance at her screen. Her browser is open to a Google Street View of a crop circle. I very slowly sit down in the lime-green plastic chair and tremble at the thought of where this is going.

· · ·

"I'll be honest with you. I was pretty intrigued by your research query. I haven't done much of that in the last few years, changing interests and such, but can you tell me what the specifics are so I can see if I can help you out?"

I look around me. A group of sticky ninth graders has just poured through the door. Beside us is a mom with a baby in a stroller and two near-identical female employees are running the shop. An instrumental synthesizer and flute rendition of "Take My

Breath Away" replaces Céline. These are not really the environmental conditions I would choose for disclosing my life story.

"I was hoping you could look into my parents—"

"Your parents?"

"Yes. They're dead . . . AIDS."

"Who raised you?"

"My grandmother."

"Where is she?"

"Inglewood Park Cemetery."

"Oh god, I'm so sorry! When?"

"June."

"Of this year?"

She moves like an insect or bird—everything is tight and on the verge of exploding. She keeps her hands knotted together in front of her, while her left thigh bounces up and down like she's a fourteen-year-old with ADHD. Her eyes are open, clear, and dart between me and her laptop screen.

"So your parents passed away and I'm guessing you don't have anyone around who can fill in the blanks. Like where they worked, where they lived before getting married, those types of things?"

"Yes. Right. My parents had friends, but after they died they just kind of vanished . . ."

"Were your parents native Angelenos?" She leans into the Spanish pronunciation quite hard.

"Belfast, and San Juan, Puerto Rico."

"Fuck! I thought you were going to say, like, Fresno and Pasadena."

I take a quick glance at the ninth graders and the mom to see if the "Fuck" gave anyone pause. Fortunately, everyone seems wrapped up in their own little universes.

"And AIDS?"

"My dad slept around a lot . . . but . . . who knows? I don't have details on any of this."

"What about you?"

"How do you mean?"

"Well, I'm assuming you're HIV-negative, but you could have gotten it, couldn't you? Your mom might have got infected while pregnant—or before."

The air between us chills.

"I'm sorry," she says. "It's just, this is what I would want to know if I was in your position. The other stuff, old apartments, old spouses, who cares?"

"It helps me fill in a picture."

She sighs and looks directly at me. "You want to know if they were good people? If they did nice things for each other, for friends, if they were well regarded, blah, blah, blah."

"Yes. And there's something else."

I give her my dad's name and she googles him right then and there. A flood rises in my chest of something black, like tar. I start to sink into it, and my vision tightly narrows. My breath turns into something I have to think about so it will continue to happen, but underneath this drowning sensation is pure anger: I refuse to lose consciousness in an establishment called It's Boba Time. I keep watching the second hand go round on the giant wall clock shaped like a strawberry. Even though I see it rotating through its circuit I have no idea how long this pause has been. Then I realize Katherine has been narrating her search finds and I snap back to attention.

"People think your dad is still alive. They think he faked his own death—"

"You couldn't fake the kind of dying I saw."

"Of course, but it's weird people would think that. I mean, what's the story there?"

"I don't know. It's the internet."

She nods and shrugs. I nod and shrug. She stares into her screen. I stare into my hands.

"Let me see what I can do for you. I'm sure I can dig around and find out some answers, besides, I've done stranger things before, and I like you. Your heart is in the right place."

"How can you tell something like that?"

"I'm also a psychic."

Driving south in my lilac Mini Cooper I realize I forgot to ask her essential questions such as her daily rate. I send her a text requesting a quote and all I get back in response is "Don't worry about it now. All will be revealed soon," followed by a winking emoji.

NOT REWRITE YOU

It is hard not to let something rewrite you. The force of a thing can shred every cell of your nervous system and turn you into something you were not meant to be. Trauma breaks the tethers to gravity, sends you reeling into electric black space. And that could be your life, drifting along that vector extending endlessly through frozen clouds of dust.

The problem is that your life can be rewritten, but the part of you that retains your original (genetic?) imprint cannot. You become a mix of two timelines, a Before and an After, and they spiral around each other in a continuous friction. But at the end of the

241

day you have a choice: do you want to be the story of trauma, or do you want to write your own story? So, I'm writing—

You can do it too.

FLICKERING SCREENS

The multiplexes we used to go to back then have closed or been rebranded as new luxury chains. These theaters, sprinkled around the South Bay and Santa Monica, are still landmarks in my mind, despite their current mutations. Right on Pacific Coast Highway there used to be an AMC on the highest floor of a stucco plaza. Its neon marquee curved above a pair of long escalators that led straight down to the sidewalk. Just a few blocks from the beach, the place had an oceanic vibe, and the walls were painted the pink of a seashell's interior. The surrounding businesses were a rotating blend of waxing salons, frozen yogurt shops, doctors' offices, and surf boutiques. Some spaces remained perpetually vacant, which is probably why the whole plaza was foreclosed. It sat empty for a time, encircled by a chain-link fence, but then was bought, gutted, and transformed into sleek offices covered in tinted glass. Nearby was the Bijou, a small art house with two screens. The paint on its southern side peeled off in chips, and parts of the flower molding had been smeared by constant exposure to sea salt. The whiteness of its two stories, coupled with the dehydration of its wear and tear, gave the impression of a crumbling wedding cake. Today it is a Chase Bank branch with flat-screen monitors advertising credit card APRs in liquid crystal displays. Another theater was housed in a former bowling alley, which retained much of its original seventies décor, from the carpet to the signage. Because of this, it ran as a discount shop, showing blockbusters for three dollars months after their release.

I know these places have been erased, but sometimes I swear I can feel their screens still standing, still active, with the shadows of all the films they've ever played moving across them in the dark. Their stories continue, gliding over one another in an epic loop of superimposition, while the world outside changes: trees grow and their roots displace chunks of sidewalk, teenagers become activists or social media stars, cars become mildly electric, phone booths disappear, information gets stored in clouds, temperatures rise, but the films just keep on playing. Their silver imprints continue to linger, becoming encased in a new geology we have no words for yet, like glowing caves hidden within cities, caves of crystals.

END OF TRANSMISSION

The WHO validates Cuba as the first nation in the world to end mother-to-child transmission of HIV in 2015. This form of viral spread is considered eliminated when the rates of newborn infection no longer statistically register as a public health issue: "In the case of HIV, this is defined as fewer than 2 in every 100 babies born to women with HIV." Early preventative measures such as testing and universal healthcare are cited as the reasons for this success.

PHOTOS OF EMPTY ROADS

In the library, I open a book with pictures of empty roads. I turn a page and remember an old feeling. I flow inside asphalt lanes piercing pale desert sands, and the hairs on my arms prick up as if activated by an arid breeze.

AUTOCOMPLETE

If you google "is the internet," the top three autocompletes are (today):

- down
- down in my area
- working

TALK TO TEXT

She calls me from the car, a pearlescent Cabrio convertible, like the one from the commercial. The mini-narrative of its hipster dream life is etched into my memory: young, perfect, alive, four friends drive alongside a moonlit body of water—the Pacific—while Nick Drake's "Pink Moon" plays in the background. I think now of those faces, circa 2000, and the stars shimmering above them as Katherine gives me a status report. "Hey! So, so sorry to call you from the road. Things have been absolutely cray-zee today. I thought I would be at my destination by now."

"That's okay. Don't worry about it."

"I might lose you when I go into the canyon, but if I do I'll call you right back when I'm on the other side."

"It's all fine."

I scheduled this call through an unnecessarily protracted email exchange to pinpoint a date and time we could both speak distraction-free. Now I'm hearing the actual wind rush through her hair. As she details the "insanity" of her morning, I give up and slice a lime for a gin and tonic. I reach for the Tanqueray in the cupboard then approximate a 50ml pour into a Garfield mug. So far, all I've been following of this conversation are the hisses of static, though the odd words like "peyote" and "briefcase" have escaped. I top off my drink with some flat Fever-Tree, take a swig, and finally interject, "Katherine, I was wondering if you have any information for me because if not—the connection is really bad—"

"Yes, sorry, yes. I tracked down some details about your father but before I go into all of that, I want to make sure you feel comfortable—"

And then she's gone. In my mind's eye I see her convertible on a thread of road dwarfed by ancient red rocks. My face starts to burn. I down half my drink.

My phone vibrates. The message reads, "Hey! So I lost you obvs!!! Monkey face buried in hands."

Is this a sentence?

I text back, "?"

"Oh. HA. HA. I am doing talk to text because I can't call and my voice memos isn't working."

It takes me a minute to figure out how to respond. I don't want this girl texting while she's driving so for the first time in my life, I attempt a voice memo. I whisper into the phone, "Cool. No prob," like it is a human ear.

A message comes back. "I found some documents your dad shuffle house."

"Sorry, come again?" I record and send.

"No. Not shuffle house," comes back. Then, "I said: SHUFFLE HOUSE."

"What are you saying, Katherine? What is 'Shuffle House'?"

"HA. HA. That is funny can't believe it corrects to Shuffle House. Have no idea where House—HA HA HA HA—"

"Can I call you later? I think the sound interference is affecting the autocorrect in a really strange way."

"No. The reception will end in muffin miles."

"Maybe you can tell me the most important thing from your investigation?"

"That's so cute, smiley face, investigation! Blushing face. Look, Heather, the thing. Oh no—one bar, breaking already?"

"What was that? What is breaking?"

"Damn. Signal is breaking. Not you. HA HA. Not you. You are fine. Okay. Do you hear me? You are so fine. You don't need any of this. Shuffle House, Shuffle, whatever—the documents will not fix. You are now smiley face."

I supply what I think are her missing words. "The past is past?" I whisper into the phone that is not a thing with blood rushing through it, but a mechanical device.

"Right! Yeah! It doesn't matter where you've come from—fuck, it's breaking—"

I cut the line, or I would have if we lived in the time when you could hang up on someone.

LIKE CANADA?

In 2015, a record-breaking seventy million photos a day are posted on Instagram. This is roughly equivalent to twice the population of Canada.

THING

You can bring someone back from the dead and fold them inside a sentence.

FIVE IMAGES OF MY PARENTS DYING OF AIDS

1. The couch is a cream color with flowers in aubergine, burgundy, and ultramarine. Thin twisting stems link them together as they branch out over the expanse of the fabric, a floral lattice binding the upholstery. Sinking into it is David. His body disintegrates into the armrests and seat cushions, merging into these structures as if his bones were liquid. Case in point, his glasses melt into the contours of his face, forcibly propping up his eyebrow ridge. He is becoming an amalgam of objects. He is becoming something other than a man. Enveloping his form is skin so wan it reminds me of fish of the deep, their scales so clear you can see their tiny, blue veins pulsing inside.

2. The nurse has delicate braids gathered together and rolled into a French twist. Four tiny gold flowers arranged in a line run parallel to it, transforming a clean and functional hairstyle into a statement. Taller than the other nurses, with the shoulders of a swimmer, she has an athlete's air, and can somehow lift Vivian in and out of hospital beds and wheelchairs without so much as breaking a sweat. It astounds me, not just her strength, but her ability to slide on latex gloves and swab raw, dripping bedsores. I watch her switch out overflowing bedpans and wonder how she does it when other people become insurance brokers or librarians. Through a doorway, I study the details of the flowers, and overhear her conversation with Nivia. She has a daughter around my age. As my eyes wander over the etched petals, I seriously consider whether I would switch places with the daughter if the laws of the universe allowed: is it harder to

watch your mother die once, or watch your mother care for the dying over and over and over again?

3. I open the front door and see Vivian stretched out on the couch in the same way David once was. A long green nightgown the texture of a sweatshirt covers the skeleton of her body. On a chair next to her is Nivia, who shoves a plastic straw between her cracked lips. Vivian is being force-fed. Her voice is gone, and so she cannot refuse to do things she does not want to do, like eat. Defeated, she accepts the straw and chokes down gruel composed of meat and veg blended together. Vivian's eyes catch me through the door, and plead in a way I have never seen before. She wants me to make it stop.

"What's going on?" I ask.

"Nothing. We are watching TV."

"What's on TV?"

"*Hill Street Blues*. It's a police detective show, so your mother will like it."

4. I wander into David's office. The venetian blinds are closed but little shafts of light escape and project onto the adjacent wall in a zebra pattern. IV stands are haphazardly scattered around the room, as are wax paper coverings for syringes. The massive hospital bed in the center of the space is empty. His body is gone. A hand wraps around my upper arm, the stray fibers of my acrylic ballet sweater pop up between the fingers. "You shouldn't be here," says the voice attached to the arm.

5. In the middle of the night she is sprawled on the floor in a puddle of urine. The bedside lamp has been switched on and the

wheelchair has been displaced from its station against the wall. I understand, from this constellation of objects, that she was trying to get to the bathroom but somehow collapsed. I ask her why she is still on the floor, and she says it is because she cannot stand up. To move her, I must engineer a solution utilizing the leverage of my nine-year-old body against nearby pieces of furniture. I troubleshoot different configurations until I land on one involving pure brute force: I swoop my upper back under her shoulder and deadlift, pressing and shifting until somehow, I get her into a sitting position on the wheelchair, but now what?

A PHOTOGRAPH NOT YET TAKEN

Three o'clock, the interior of a bar, Paris. A lone bartender wipes down the countertop in slow, methodical circles. He hums along to "'Round About Midnight." The last patron gets up to leave and drops a few coins on his table. "À bientôt, Michel," he calls out. The bartender nods, then everything is still for a moment before a breeze comes in and rustles the pages of the newspapers hung along the wall.

INFLUENCE CAMPAIGN

On January 6, 2017, US intelligence agencies confirm Russian interference in the 2016 presidential election. The main tactic of interference is determined to be an online "influence campaign," wherein the Internet Research Agency, a St. Petersburg company / troll farm, spreads disinformation across multiple social media platforms. This was accomplished through the creation of thousands of fake profiles.

GODWIN'S LAW

Godwin's Law: a facetious aphorism maintaining that as an online debate increases in length, it becomes inevitable that someone will eventually compare someone or something to Adolf Hitler or the Nazis. Also in extended use.

INTERNET CAFÉ

The last internet café on Earth, or at least what feels like it, is on Hackney Road, just north of St. Leonard's church in London. The café is actually two computer stalls separated by a sheet of cardboard in the back room of a barbershop. It used to be next door. The old orange banner is still there, advertising PRINTING, COMPUTER SERVICES, COFFEE—&—SNACK, but the front has been shuttered up and covered in a mural of graffiti for the last five years. How the migration of the café from its own space to this back room occurred is anyone's guess, but this block has always operated "independently," on the lower frequencies, so in some sense, it's not surprising at all. This is the East End, or it used to be. Now it's more home to craft beer bars and sneaker boutiques than drug deals. The barbershop itself is a new incarnation. Previously a grubby establishment, it is now a hybrid of traditional Turkish and hipster styles of grooming. The logo features two sharpened blades crossed at the hilts with a typeface that might best be described as Jack the Ripper Nouveau, as enough Ripper walking tours have used it to advertise their "evenings of thrills." Its aesthetic is clinical yet on point, with stainless-steel fixtures and black leather chairs. The only nod to sentimentality, or kitsch, is a barber's pole installed by the front entrance. Measuring less than a foot long, its red and blue stripes twirl ceaselessly within a clear plastic sheath. A placard sign in the window advertises a Bitcoin ATM, and directly underneath it, taped to the glass, is a note card with the word "internet" handwritten in black pen. To get to the internet, you walk along the gleaming white-tiled wall opposite the barbers' stations to a door with a full-length mirror on it. Under the mirror is another note card with an arrow and the phrase "@Access." If you follow the arrow, through the looking glass, you'll enter a corridor that eventually dead-ends at a curtain and bingo: you've found connectivity.

The café is run by a Chinese mother-and-son duo, and I get the impression they also live here, after hours. Two rolled-up sleeping bags and a few pillows are on an MDF shelf near the ceiling, and there are other personal traces, such as hotel slippers and melted candles, that suggest it doubles as a home. A mini fridge stocked with Coke, Red Bull, and Vita Coco coconut water sits in the corner. There's no coffee, despite its lineage as a café, but the mom will brew loose-leaf green tea and bring it to you in a cast-iron pot if you ask. The room has only one window, a skinny horizontal panel high up on one wall.

It is hard to say how many people know about this place, but there must still be demand since it endures. They also sell burner phones and international SIM cards, according to the Lebara advertisements on display. A calendar from 2011 is pinned open to June. Its image of a tropical beach is so flawless, so pristine, it looks like a Windows screen saver. No place in the world looks like this.

The son, who is twenty-two or twenty-three, sets me up at a terminal. His English is exquisitely American. He tells me he's going outside to make a call and smoke, if I need help with anything technical, but his mom can handle everything else. She nods from a stool and picks up a needlepoint. I put on a headset, log on to Skype, and then wait, glancing up at the digitally enhanced turquoise waves.

Earlier in the day, my phone met its demise. A finance bro bumped into me at Farringdon station and the angle of contact caused it to slide out of my hand and onto the tracks. Seconds later, the train arrived. The bro didn't seem to notice the collision or the phone and just kept walking, oblivious to the world and all the things in it. Most people around me averted their glances, but a few openly giggled, which caused me to turn on my heel and walk the two miles home without a single backward glance. Prior to the phone fiasco, the battery on my laptop went into sudden death mode so I brought it in for servicing. By the time 10 A.M. rolled around I was completely untethered from the world. On most days this wouldn't matter, but I had a planned Skype meeting with Katherine and the thought of trying to reschedule made my mouth fill with bile. If I wanted to speak to her today, and somewhat privately, this was the only option.

The mom brings me a pot of tea even though I haven't asked for one, and I try to catch her eye when I say thank you. Her face is kind but worn out, like it's held worry in its bones for a very long time. She looks around sixty-five or seventy, though her attire doesn't reflect this, or much about her identity. A T-shirt, sporting an illustration of Big Ben, hangs off the reed of her body, two sizes too large, and her corduroy trousers, striped and flared, would be an expensive find at any of the local vintage shops. The visual asymmetry of person and items speaks, at least to me, of survival, and Nivia comes rushing to mind but—now is not the time to get sentimental. Through a pale reflection on the monitor, I watch the mom arrange herself on the stool. I realize I'm not ready for what's about to happen. I decide to cut and run, but right as I lift my ass out of the chair, the Skype icon jumps all over the screen. By reflex, my hand clicks it, and then I'm fucked because there is Katherine, looking at me and smiling.

Behind her is an assortment of glistening fronds and other rubbery vegetation. The quality of light is unnaturally dewy and difficult to place. Her laptop is on the ground, on what appears to be sand, and she keeps bending down to it, to get more of her face in the frame, but the positioning is awkward.

"Hi there!" She waves. "How are you, what's going on, how's life—"

Her words chop into one another at such a percussive pace I wonder whether she's been microdosing a local psychotropic drug. A foam of questions bubbles up in my mind, but I manage to ask not a single one because she railroads me with intense chat about the weather, which, surprising as it sounds, momentarily normalizes the situation. I scrutinize the live feed for some clue as to her location. It could be either a Sandals All-Inclusive Resort, or a "spiritual wellness" retreat. Katherine is so odd she could be anywhere on this holiday spectrum. She could even be in LA staging the whole thing, but then, somewhere in the distance, is the wash of ocean surf. Straining to hear it, I slowly become aware that Katherine is staring at me wide-eyed in expectation. This is excruciating, so I finally lay it on her. "Look, if I knew you were traveling we could have postponed until you got back to LA—"

"Oh, that won't be for ages and besides, it is important to do things when you say you're going to do them, otherwise they never happen, at least in my humble opinion. Anyway, this trip just materialized out of the ether and I had to seize the opportunity, you know? Studying with Guru J is such an honor."

Ignoring the bit about the guru I say, "Sorry. Where are you exactly?"

"Oh! Yes! Sorry! I'm in a small village outside of Puerto Cayo, in Ecuador. Guru J is a *super*-well-regarded plant medicine doctor. I'm here learning about native plants and for some important me time—"

"Me time" is one of the worst phrases ever created.

"Mostly I document J's plant care procedures for herbs in Google Docs. Plus I try to absorb what I can about his creative process."

My head nods of its own accord, a flower bud collapsing on a stem. She continues to talk, describing rituals surrounding harvests, like plucking vines during full moons. I notice a tiny insect with a brightly colored shell make its way up her shinbone. It gingerly moves one leg at a time, trying to understand the unusual surface it finds itself on.

"You look upset," she says suddenly.

I don't want to lie, but I also don't want to lose my shit and shatter the gentle solitude of the cafe. There are mousetraps on the vinyl floor spread out like islands. I hadn't noticed them before.

"I just . . . I'm not sure I can handle whatever you are going to tell me. I'm not sure I can hear it."

"That is *so okay*. Oh my god, *of course*. Maybe you aren't ready, and we should wait. That's totally fine, sweetie."

Sweetie.

Between the two of us, it might be hard to say who's the bigger fool, but I'm betting it's me.

"What you found, is it awful?"

We look at each other and I can actively sense her arranging words, as if they were objects of mass and density.

"It is nearly impossible to say from what I've captured online to know if your father was truly motivated by hate or attention. Sooo many people get into controversial material because the kerfuffle surrounding it becomes intoxicating. It generates the sensation of power, but it's not *real* power, you know? I mean, look at Kanye, look at Damien Hirst, even Julian Assange. Are they wackadoodles or deeply strategic? I have no idea if your father was a revisionist, a racist, a white supremacist, or mentally ill. Maybe he just enjoyed being a provocateur, or maybe, it was about survival. Maybe the only way out of a doomed existence in Belfast was to join the National Front. As a young, handsome man in that circle, he probably would have garnered a lot of attention, and access to levels of society otherwise unavailable to him—"

"You don't need to rationalize his position."

"I'm not rationalizing his position, because there is no reason in any of this. People are messy. We don't know why we do most of what we do most of the time. Our internal vision only goes so far, even for a person like Guru J. So yeah, maybe your dad thought the Holocaust was a hoax, but did he teach *you* the lie? So, okay, he aggressively denied the murder of six million people, but what if he was actually kind to the pizza delivery guy? The mailman? The dry cleaner? What if he made people around him feel human in his day-to-day existence, and what if one of those people didn't put a bullet in their own face because your father said 'Hello' and 'Thank you' to them? How do you judge him then? If he appeared one way, but acted another?"

"Honestly, all of this is entirely speculative, and I have no memory of him ever being nice to anyone—not that that would excuse any of this—"

"But you weren't indoctrinated—"

"I was just a little kid and he thought I was dumb as a doornail, so there wouldn't be much point."

"There is definitely a point if you believe a certain thing to be The Truth."

I drink some tea, take a brief glance at the mom. It's hard to say how much of this she's getting, the video, my responses. Fortunately, the running water and deep laughter from the barber's creates a layer of sound that makes me feel partially insulated.

Katherine keeps speaking to me, but about what I cannot say. Her voice mutates into the scrape of sand and the rush of distant tides. I think very intensely of the whiskey on the top shelf of my cabinet and my eyes sink through the screen, examining everything more pointedly than before. One of the plants on her left shoulder has deep red veins spreading through it. The sand contains pebbles, most of them gray, and a few miniature seashells with impossibly refined edges. A single line running from Katherine's hairline down to her left eyebrow disrupts her otherwise smooth face. The shadows in the frame change, become drier, and less infused with equatorial tonalities. The sun must be moving. I try to listen to what she says but my brain is running interference, tearing her words apart, making them indecipherable. There is nothing to hold on to, save the technology of recorded light beamed across space and arriving on my screen as glowing bits of data that form a person. A person who knows my name and is speaking to me now.

I move the mouse to end the call, but Katherine juts in, "I know you're doing all this because you want someone to tell you whether or not your dad was a bad man, but I'm not sure I can find badness or, even a man. I'm not sure anyone can. I just pick up the traces and give them to you. That's it, okay? There's nothing else anyone can do."

"I get it."

She waves goodbye and ends the call. I hang up the headset on the corner of the monitor and stare at the screen for a few seconds before putting my head on the laminate table. It feels so cool and sturdy I just stay there. After a few minutes I feel something land on my shoulder. It feels like a hand, but the touch of it is so gentle I'm positive I'm imagining it, except—I remember I'm in public, so the hand *could* be real. I sit straight up and there is the mom holding a few tissues. I touch my cheek. There are tears all over it.

I try to say something, excuse myself, apologize, but all I can see are the echoes of Nivia cast over this woman's stature. I start to say, "My grandma, my grandma—"

"She went home?"

"Home?"

She points to the calendar photo of the white beach and palm trees, and for a split second all the wires in my brain hysterically seize. I think she means that Nivia has "gone home" to a tropical paradise well beyond this world.

LIKE CICERO, IN HIS LIBRARY

I knew all of this was doomed to fail. Knew it before I got on a plane, made a call, typed things into a search engine, because none of it was real. What I mean is: if you want The Truth, or at least the version of it you can live with, you have to find it yourself.

CRISPR BABIES

In November 2018, a story from China made international headlines: twin girls were born with a genetic resistance to HIV infection. Their genomes had been modified at the embryonic phase with CRISPR technology to eradicate the potential for the disease. Since CRISPR's emergence in 2005, scientists have struggled to contain its genuinely awesome power, researching at a snail's pace out of reverence for the numerous ethical concerns genetic editing raises. Basic clinical trials involving mice and other "lesser" creatures were just beginning in labs around the world. Experimentation on humans, let alone human embryos, was nowhere in sight. When the story broke, experts ranging from philosophers to biologists called the action "unconscionable," "monstrous," "irresponsible," "dangerous," and "crazy" in the press.

Under the guise of providing fertility treatments, biophysicist He Jiankui of the Southern University of Science and Technology, Shenzhen, China, modified the embryos of seven couples. These couples shared an emotional and medical vulnerability: the male partners were all HIV-positive. The objective of He's work was "to offer couples affected by HIV a chance to have a child that might be protected from a similar fate," but this motivation was shadowy at best. As the effects of gene editing on human biology are completely unknown, the risk versus reward of this scenario could not be determined. As Julian Savulescu, a professor of practical ethics at Oxford University, explained to *The Guardian,* "There are many effective ways to prevent HIV in healthy individuals: for example, protected sex. And there are effective treatments if one does contract it. This experiment exposes healthy normal children to risks of gene editing for no real necessary benefit."

On a purely scientific level, He used CRISPR to eliminate the CCR5 gene in the embryos. CCR5 codes for a protein that sits on the surface of white blood cells, which HIV virions use as a gateway to penetrate cells. If this protein does not exist in the body, infection becomes impossible . . . Unless, of course, the host has been exposed to a *different* strain of HIV that hacks into cells via a *different* protein. Alas, He's CRISPR modification only protects the twins from one viral strain of HIV, if it has even been successful at that. Other than He's own proclamations, there's no way to truly verify if the twins are in fact HIV-immune.

Research on CCR5 is still new. Over the last decade the protein has caught the eye of medical researchers working in the fields of memory and stroke rehabilitation, particularly at UCLA: "In an attempt to understand what influences memory formation and learning in the brain, a group of researchers at UCLA found that lowering the levels of CCR5 production enhanced both learning and memory formation." It was also discovered that "people missing at least one copy of the [CCR5] gene seem to go further in school, suggesting a possible role in everyday intelligence." This proposition was tested in 2016 when researchers sought to determine which genetic modifications could make mice "smarter." They concluded that removing the CCR5 gene had a strong effect in sharpening rodent intelligence.

He was reportedly aware of these studies before proceeding with his own experimentation, which begs the question: was he trying to build a line of HIV-resistant people, or one of higher IQs? The general consensus is that HIV was, in this case, a Trojan horse.

CONSISTENT WITH ACTUAL DNA DATA

In 2019, researchers at Los Alamos National Laboratory confirm that computer simulations can accurately predict the spread of HIV through populations. The study involved creating simulations of viral spread and cross-referencing the computer-generated results against hard data stored in a global, public HIV database. According to an article in *Science Daily*, the simulation results were "robust" and "consistent with actual DNA data," which means this technology can be adapted to "predict the patterns of other rapidly evolving infectious diseases."

MATTERS INTO MY OWN HANDS

There comes a moment when, if you want your life to go somewhere, you have to take it into your own hands, so I made my fingers reach across the keyboard. I typed. I clicked. I entered. One last Google search. The final goodbye—

THINGS I KNOW ABOUT MY FATHER

1. Born in Belfast

2. Died when I was seven

3. Was incredibly tall

4. Liked to dance in the living room with me to traditional Irish music

5. Wore glasses

6. Rode a bicycle in shorts

7. Enjoyed New York–style cheesecake

8. Never expressed any controversial or strange political views directly to me

9. Died in excruciating agony

THINGS THE INTERNET
SAYS ABOUT MY FATHER

1. Born in Belfast in 1952

2. Died of viral pneumonia caused by AIDS at age thirty-nine

3. Served as the director of the Institute for Historical Review and editor in chief of its newsletter from 1978 to 1980. The IHR claims it does not deny the Holocaust but questions the dominant narrative of its history. The Southern Poverty Law Center regards the IHR as a hate group.

4. Married to a "non-white woman"

5. Was a neo-Nazi, an atheist, and a "closeted homosexual"—because: AIDS

6. Was anti-Nazi, anti-establishment, an atheist, and a "closeted homosexual"—because: AIDS

7. Generally described as "eccentric"

8. On June 7, 1987, he was thrown into a plate glass window. The attack may or may not have been perpetrated by his ideological counterpart/nemesis of the Jewish Defense League.

9. The end of his *Los Angeles Times* obituary reads: "McCalden remained in the news, branding 'The Diary of Anne Frank' as 'revisionist literature' and offering libraries copies of books he said refuted the Holocaust."

WORDS I PIN MY LIFE TO

"How wonderful it is that nobody need wait a single
moment before starting to improve the world!"
— *Tales from the Secret Annex*
by ANNE FRANK

ALL I KNOW IS

You have a story and I have a story and they are not the same story. This is necessary, otherwise how else would we evolve?

THE LONDON PATIENT

At the 2019 Conference on Retroviruses and Opportunistic Infections, the case of the "London Patient" is presented. It bears a striking resemblance to that of the famed Berlin patient from 2008. After being diagnosed with Hodgkin's lymphoma, the HIV-positive London patient endured a round of chemotherapy that decimated his immune system. He then received a bone marrow transplant from a donor with a genetic mutation that confers resistance to HIV infection. As the patient's immune system had to be rebuilt from scratch, it adopted the characteristics of the donor's marrow, including the crucial genetic mutation. When the treatment was completed, the London patient ceased his antiviral regime. Twenty-nine months later, extensive testing revealed no active viral infection, heralding him as the second person in history to be cured of HIV.

CONTAGION

There's information on a screen. There are memories. Neither constitutes a narrative, or a presence, except you feel it just the same.

RADIO CITY MUSIC HALL

The first time I saw Radio City Music Hall was by accident. I was on a long, aimless walk with my eyes fixed on the sidewalk when I lifted my chin for some reason and there it was. The sight of it burned through my mental haze and suddenly I became vividly aware of existing. Radio City had been built into my mind through so many secondhand sources, I had categorized it more as a fiction and less a physical location that I might one day be able to visit. Now I was colliding with it, unexpectedly, and reeling; the intersection of matter and myth induced a vertiginous thrill completely unknown to me. The ground lurched. I laughed, and then I saw

Nivia as a young woman exit the building. The pleats of her gray wool skirt stretched open as she pushed through the lobby door, and promptly accordioned back together, swishing a bit once she was out on the street. As she reached into the black pocketbook caught in the crook of her elbow, I glimpsed her face made up in lipstick and blush. Her expression reminded me of a sprig of rosemary swirling in a champagne coupe. She was amused, gleeful; she slipped on a pair of white gloves before turning up Sixth Avenue.

I followed the mirage uptown for blocks, until the shout of a hot dog vendor and a chorus of fire truck sirens dissolved it. But I kept walking into the night, past bodegas and art galleries, diners, perfume stores, restaurants, dog grooming parlors, and pencil towers. I kept walking past the textures and histories of all these buildings, only thinking of Nivia sitting in the dark and watching luminous faces blown up like gods on the Radio City screen.

UNIVERSAL PROPERTIES

What if "the truth" of healing is simply movement and time?

WILDERNESS

I look at the blank page on my desk and think: Finally, my friend. Here we are at last. Just the two of us. Listening to music.

Everything else—the bamboo shutters of the room, the scent of freshly cut geraniums in the air, a segment of light coming in from underneath a door—fades out. I lose my face. There's nothing to look at. Somewhere, over in the corner, is where I leave my second skin, twisted like a wet towel. Somewhere, in an electronic bank account, the accumulation of blood, sweat, and tears is summarized in zeroes and ones. But now, we can lose track of all that. Now we can just be a pen moving across paper and feel something so delicate and precise all other sensations cease to exist.

A wolf howls at the moon, maybe, somewhere in another country. Beyond these windows, the wilderness, beyond the wilderness, the world, beyond the world, the universe.

ONE HUNDRED CENTURIES

In a 2019 paper published in *Nature,* Google announces that its quantum computer, called Sycamore, has achieved "quantum supremacy," a state "when a quantum computer can perform a calculation that a traditional computer can't complete within its lifetime." Purportedly, Sycamore only needs two hundred seconds to finish a highly esoteric task that would take "a state-of-the-art classical supercomputer" somewhere in the vein of ten thousand years to resolve.

THE DETECTIVE'S WISDOM

The detective already knows the pearls are fakes, and the negatives (of the naked heiress) are stowed behind the potted ferns in the foyer. He knows the blackmailer is the jealous husband, and that the "missing" sister is either dead already or never existed in the first place. The detective already knows whatever you're looking for is a) not *actually* what you're looking for and b) gone for good.

Most of all, he knows none of it matters. Your mystery is but a smudge on the lens of time—and guess what, lady? That's just the way it is.

CAVE OF CRYSTALS

In a cave in the Mexican state of Chihuahua, there are thousands of crystals that measure over thirty feet long and weigh over fifty tons. Their translucent beams shoot out of the limestone walls and crisscross the cave's chamber like frozen searchlights. They seem to glow. In photographs, people in hazmat suits standing next to them resemble ants and other tiny insects.

The cave was discovered in 2000 when miners working for Industrias Peñoles were excavating a tunnel. Ancient volcanic activity is thought to have incited the folds and crevices of land that formed this space eight hundred feet below the ground. Its isolated nature and unique interior properties were such that selenite was able to grow to epic proportions. Selenite is a type of gypsum, a calcium sulfate dihydrate most commonly used in fertilizer and chalk. Another variety of it is alabaster, which means the sculpted rippling torsos of antiquity are of the same lineage as the beasts of this cavern.

The miners were the first humans to enter this cave.

It is nearly impossible to imagine a location on Earth that no human has stood in and breathed, a place where no one has taken a selfie to say: Look, I was *there*. All the cave knows is the intimate passage of geological time, the movement of heat, water, and minerals, and their transference of energy. A silence enters me when I try to conjure the sense of such a place; my blood grows still at the thought of it.

Scientists eventually secured access to the cave and took samples of the crystals and groundwater to study back in their labs. Dr. Curtis Suttle of the University of British Columbia analyzed the contents of a single drop of water and found within it two hundred million viruses, none of which had ever been encountered before.

AT THE ROYALE

The brushed steel doors of the elevator slide open and inside is a drag queen leaning on the railing. There is so much of her, I can't take her in with one glance. Between the sculpted hair, ice-pick heels, tulle, and faux fur, each part of her only materializes as a close-up. I try to collage the details together, but my senses are blotto, so she remains a cloud of rhinestones and nylons shimmering under a grid of LEDs. In my experience, a drag queen showing up in one's night sometime after 1 A.M. is either a harbinger of joy or catastrophe.

"Well, you getting in?" she says in a Southern drawl.

I take a step inside and the doors swiftly shut at my back. Encountering this sugarplum vision when I was anticipating an empty cubicle of space completely disorients me. YSL Black Opium hangs in the air.

"What floor you going to?"

I hadn't thought about that yet. I just found myself at the hotel elevator bank and it seemed natural to hit the up arrow. Panic must be swirling over my face because she says gently, "How 'bout penthouse? Top floor?"

I nod my head, slowly. Penthouse sounds good. She extracts a key card from her bra and taps it on the sensor. Her face is extraordinarily painted, with planes and shadows carved into it like a pastoral landscape. Slight marks of tarnish are visible though, most certainly evidence of a long night of performing in the burlesque club in the basement. A tick of purple lipstick reaches down toward her chin, and a streak of black eyeliner loses the plot of her bottom lid. Sweat glistens along her hairline. As I study the beads of sweat on her brow, I realize that she's looking at me.

"Honey, you mind taking a quick picture of me right now? I'm enjoying all these reflections."

"Uhhh. Okay. Sure."

"No flash, baby. Here."

She hands me her iPhone X and then drapes herself, like a heroine from a Pre-Raphaelite painting, over the railing. She elongates her neck and arches it backward before turning to look at the camera. Then she gives a long, luxurious bat of the lashes. "Okay. Ready," she says.

The walls are full-length smoky mirrors so her magnificence, along with my dull appearance, extends outward in a thousand directions.

"I'm in the photo. Is that okay?"

"Sure is, but take the thing before the ride is over."

I take a few, zoom in, zoom out, landscape, portrait, and hand her the phone just as the doors crack open. The Queen tells me to follow her and we walk down a long corridor that seems to keep bending and switching directions. The lighting is dim, coming from tiny antique sconces on the walls. On closer examination the sconces seem to have angel faces. I look down and away from them. Burgundy hexagons outlined in brown cover the carpet in an offset honeycomb pattern that hurts my brain. I keep trying to psychically realign them against their background of burnt orange, but it unnerves me. The pattern increases the feeling of wandering in a labyrinth. I lose track as to whether we are passing the same baroque-looking table with an overflowing vase of peonies, or whether there are multiple tables and multiple vases. The strange and decadent ambiance seems designed to induce a sense of intoxication. The thing is, I'm already three sheets so all of this quickly unravels to the point where a minotaur in quiet pursuit of us is not out of the realm of possibility. Fortunately, the Queen pushes open what looks like a linen closet and leads us up a narrow staircase to fresh air.

The Thames, a glistening wire, twists sixty floors beneath us, and the lights of the city fracture the night into a thousand untold stories never to be thought of again after this moment.

The Queen waves me over. It seems I've been staring into the smoldering windows of an office building for longer than acceptable. I navigate across the roof debris, lightly stepping between rotting cardboard and shards of glass. The Queen stands in a pile of cigarette butts. The secret staff smoking spot, I imagine.

"Bar staff comes up here on breaks," she says, reading my mind. "But, I'm done for the night. Last show just finished."

She passes me a cigarette and lights it with a match, then we just stand there smoking in silence, looking over London Town spread wide open beneath us. There doesn't seem to be anything to say. Smoke gets pulled down into the lungs and exhaled in ribbons. The cigarettes turn into ash, the ash blows away. Fresh cigarettes are lit, and the beast of the city in all its heartbreak and history is swallowed in a single glance. This must be why people climb mountains.

"It is so strange," she says, "we can't choose when we come into this world or when we leave it, but we have to choose every little thing in between. Every damn second in between, you have to choose to be something—"

"Or what?"

"Or else you're nothing, baby. Time's gonna sweep you right up if you don't make yourself into something . . . I mean, we're all dust in the end, but until then you can be more."

I notice she's squinting one eye and blinking the other rapidly. She peels off one of her lashes and puts it in her palm. It looks like an exotic caterpillar until its mate joins it, and suddenly it's a thing with wings that she blows off into the air with a soft "Bye, bye." The level of conversation is so instantly and unexpectedly real, an anchor drops inside my chest. This is how I wish it could be with people. I watch the paper of my cigarette slowly recede.

"Do you think people do that? Get there, I mean?"

She takes a long drag, hieroglyphic-like lipstick traces remaining on the filter. "I think people let things get in the way. They let things rewrite them. Pain mostly. You gotta broken heart 'cause he left you or she died or this, that, whatever, the pain can rewrite your entire system. Make you into something you weren't meant to be and then, that's the story of your life and that's a shame, baby. Damn shame. That's letting pain write you. Put it like this: you wanna be the story of heartache or you wanna write your own story? Don't look so sad, baby. You gonna figure it out."

"How do you know that?"

The Queen looks at me and kills her cigarette with the lethal blade of her heel.

"A little bird told me. A little flyby, butterfly. She told me to look for you."

"Ah, I didn't take you for a sweet talker!"

Then she roars, volcanic laughter erupting from her throat and into the night and so I laugh too, until tears streak my whole face.

"Anyone who is polite enough to listen to this old queen ramble into the early morning hours is a real person, so don't be giving up just yet. A friend of mine, Charlotte Hibiscus, is in the hospital right now waiting for a kidney. She can still walk a bit, so every day she does her face, puts a wig on, and she shuffles through the ward draggin' her IV. Honey looks like a nightmare in a hospital gown and violet eye shadow, but she visits the other patients. Makes them laugh, you know, still doing parts of her act . . . The kidney probably ain't gonna come but that doesn't stop her from being *her*. You get it? She ain't stopping. You get what I'm saying to you?"

"Yeah. I think so."

"Of course you do. Now, let's take a picture so you don't forget."

I think she means a picture of the two of us, a selfie of some sort, but she arranges me solo on a bucket à la Venus sprouting up out of the clamshell.

"Honey, don't be scared, I gotta use the flash up here. I know, I know. It's okay. Flash ain't nothing to be afraid of unless you're indoors. Okay, now you gotta lean into the left hip. No honey, *lean*, really lean. Why you not leaning? You have bursitis in your hip, girl? Then come on, *sink* into it. SINK!"

I'm giggling so much I just melt onto the bucket in slow motion and prop my back against the low safety wall. I take a quick peek over my shoulder down at the river and the lights and I try to put it all inside me so I might be able to glow, at least for the photograph. The Queen then snaps her fingers and I whip back around to face the camera.

"Smile, darling. You look beautiful."

ACKNOWLEDGMENTS

Of all the pages in this book, this is the one I longed to write the most. You can't get very far in a life like mine without encouragement and love, and I've often dreamt of a circumstance that would allow me to issue a record of thanks to all the people who have genuinely stood by me for all these years. With this being said, let me begin by thanking my teachers, who have quite literally given me everything:

To Dr. Lucy Soutter, without whom I might have never seriously picked up a pen; to Michael Turco for showing me what it is to live life as if it were art; to Summer Lee Rhatigan for repairing my nervous system through classical ballet; to Susan Butler for numerous analytical conversations over espressos in East London; to Marian Kliger, who first illuminated the relationship between art and society to me as a shy fifteen-year-old. My world, Marian, has never been the same, and only continues to evolve in complexity and beauty because of the foundation you gave me.

My most heartfelt thanks to the readers of the first iteration of this book: Drew Jerrison, Katie Daubs, Patrick Taylor, and

Gabrielle Zucker. Beyond providing insightful critique, each of you offered the most potent feedback possible: keep going.

Major thanks to the Banff Centre for Arts and Creativity and the Mahler & LeWitt Studios, which provided space and time to reflect on language. Guy Robertson: your generous thoughts and aperitivi will never be forgotten.

Special thanks to the former children's librarians of the El Segundo Public Library, Sindee Pickens, Carol Craft, and Roger Kelly, who gave me my first safe refuge: stories.

I am grateful to the cohort of writers I met at Tin House, especially Cass Lewis, Jackie Domenus, and Gabriel Stein-Bodenheimer. Your words and life experiences have driven me to ask more of life and words.

To Cyrus Dunham, for the all-important lesson of sculpting memoir from the parts of self we keep "out of frame," or diving into the fire rather than being ashamed of it.

To Megan Kurashige, for being an exquisite human.

To Bert Henert for generosity, love, and a place to call home.

To Reena Esmail, for being my soul-tuning fork.

To Joshua Leon, for tracking down the origins of a crucial quote, and for many lovely conversations about art and comedy.

To Virginia Fung and Steve Sunseri, for always having my back—and laughing with me about everything.

To Parisa Ebrahimi and David Ebershoff, for incisive feedback, gentle guidance, and unwavering support. Thank you for seeing value in my work and giving me the chance to share it with others.

Thank you to the teams of Fitzcarraldo Editions (particularly Joely Day and Clare Bogen) and Hogarth Books for this incredible ride.

To Jacques Testard, words are failing me here, but thank you for changing my life.

Lastly, I am no one without my dear and electric friends: Madhur Anand, Nick Arvanitis, Camden Avery, Melissa Bohlsen, Andrew Chan, Karen Chan-Morales, Kris Clarke, Miguele de Quadros-Sherry, Elizabeth De Witt, Mercedes Gilliom, Douglas Glover, Lou Grantham, Osha Hanfling, Sara Hibbert, Ruth Hogan, Mette Slot Johnsen, Sophie Kalkreuth, Lee Kvern, Lauren Morrow, Jesse Rimler, Crystal Rivette, Christy Saville, Elida Schogt, Olivia Wright, the café at Rough Trade East, and SFG, who taught me to never settle.

BIBLIOGRAPHY

BOOKS

Aristotle, *The Poetics of Aristotle,* trans. S. H. Butcher (London: Macmillan, 1895).

Baldwin, Rosecrans, *Everything Now: Lessons from the City-State of Los Angeles* (New York: MCD, a division of Farrar, Straus and Giroux, 2021).

Biss, Eula, *On Immunity: An Inoculation* (London: Fitzcarraldo Editions, 2015).

Burroughs, William, *The Ticket That Exploded* (London: Fourth Estate, 2010).

Carson, Anne, *Men in the Off Hours* (New York: Knopf Doubleday, 2009).

Chandler, Raymond, *The Big Sleep* (London: Penguin Books Ltd., 2011).

———, *The Long Good-bye* (London: Penguin Books Ltd., 2010).

Cicero, *Letters to Atticus, Volume I,* trans. and ed. D. R. Shackleton Bailey (Cambridge, Mass.: Harvard University Press, 1999).

Crawford, Dorothy H., *Viruses: A Very Short Introduction* (Oxford: Oxford University Press, 2011).

Geary, James, *I Is an Other: The Secret Life of Metaphor and How It Shapes the Way We See the World* (New York: Harper Perennial, 2012).

Lakoff, George, and Mark Johnson, *Metaphors We Live By* (Chicago: University of Chicago Press, 2003).

Maxwell, William, *So Long, See You Tomorrow* (London: Penguin Books Ltd., 2012).

Nicol, Bran, *The Private Eye: Detectives in the Movies* (London: Reaktion Books, 2013).

Rilke, Rainer Maria, *The Notebooks of Malte Laurids Brigge,* trans. Michael Hulse (London: Penguin Classics, 2009).

Ruefle, Mary, *Madness, Rack, and Honey: Collected Lectures* (Seattle: Wave Books, 2012).

Tokarczuk, Olga, *Flights,* trans. Jennifer Croft (London: Fitzcarraldo Editions, 2017).

ARTICLES AND JOURNALS

Anderson, Thomas F., "Electron Microscopy of Phages," in *Phage and the Origins of Molecular Biology,* by Gunther Stent, James D. Watson, and J. Cairns, ed. by Gunther S. Stent and J. D. Watson, The Centennial Edition (Cold Spring Harbor, N.Y.: Cold Spring Harbor Press, 1966), pp. 63–78.

"Anne Frank," Wikiquote, https://en.wikiquote.org/wiki/Anne_Frank.

Aristotle, "Metaphor is halfway between the unintelligible and the commonplace," https://quotefancy.com/quote/767801/Aristotle-Metaphor-is-halfway-between-the-unintelligible-and-the-commonplace.

Arute, Frank, Kunal Arya, Ryan Babbush, et al., "Quantum Supremacy Using a Programmable Superconducting Processor," *Nature* (October 23, 2019): 574, https://www.nature.com/articles/s41586-019-1666-5.

Berners-Lee, Tim, "Information Management: A Proposal," (March 1989, May 1990), https://www.w3.org/History/1989/proposal.html.

Bowers, John, Clare Stanton, and Jonathan Zittrain, "What the Ephemerality of the Web Means for Your Hyperlinks," *Columbia Journalism Review*

(May 21, 2021), https://www.cjr.org/analysis/linkrot-content-drift
-new-york-times.php.

Care, Christina, "Haunted by Your Own Ghosts: Dealing with the Past
and Recurring Memories: Moving Beyond Shame and Trauma,"
(May 3, 2019), https://christinacare.medium.com/haunted-by-your
-own-ghosts-dealing-with-recurring-memories-a9319805b2e9.

"Culture," Merriam-Webster.com, https://www.merriam-webster.com
/dictionary/culture.

Dafoe, Taylor, "A Laptop Infected with Six of the World's Most Dangerous Computer Viruses Is Up for Auction. The Bid Is Now More
Than $1.2 Million," *Artnet* (May 22, 2019), https://news.artnet.com
/market/malware-artwork-goes-to-auction-1554505.

eBay News Team, "A Note from eBay's Founder on Our 22nd Anniversary,"
(September 5, 2017), https://www.ebayinc.com/stories/news/a-note
-from-ebays-founder.

Ellroy, James, "The Great Right Place: James Ellroy Comes Home," *Los Angeles Times* (July 30, 2006), https://www.latimes.com/archives/la
-xpm-2006-jul-30-tm-ellroy31-story.html.

"Emotion," Merriam-Webster.com, https://www.merriam-webster.com
/dictionary/emotion.

Gómez-Gardeñes, J., L. Lotero, S. N. Taraskin, and F. J. Pérez-Reche, "Explosive Contagion in Networks," *Scientific Reports* vol. 6 (January 28,
2016), https://www.nature.com/articles/srep19767.

Guynup, Sharon, "Is Seeing Believing?," *Scientific American* Special Editions
22 (September 1, 2013), https://www.scientificamerican.com/article
/is-seeing-believing/.

Hester, Jessica, "The Phone Booth for Japanese Mourners," *Bloomberg* (January 10, 2017), https://www.bloomberg.com/news/articles/2017-01
-10/japan-s-wind-phone-is-a-site-to-mediate-on-life-and-loss.

"HIV," World Health Organization, https://www.who.int/health-topics
/hiv-aids.

"HIV Virus Spread, Evolution Studied Through Computer Modeling," *Science Daily* (November 19, 2013), https://www.sciencedaily.com/releases/2013/11/131119142232.htm.

Hjort, Jim, "Three Things You Can Do to Stop Being Haunted by Regret," https://www.jimhjort.com/articles/three-things-you-can-do-to-stop-being-haunted-by-regret.

"Internet Metaphors," Wikipedia, https://en.wikipedia.org/wiki/Internet_metaphors.

Keim, Brandon, "A Neuroscientist's Radical Theory of How Networks Become Conscious," *Wired* (November 14, 2013), https://www.wired.com/2013/11/christof-koch-panpsychism-consciousness/.

Kruger, D. H., P. Schneck, and H. R. Gelderblom, "Helmut Ruska and the Visualisation of Viruses," (May 13, 2000), http://helmut.ruska.de/?page_id=14.

Lanciani, Rodolfo, "Pagan and Christian Rome," (1892), http://penelope.uchicago.edu/Thayer/E/Gazetteer/Places/Europe/Italy/Lazio/Roma/Rome/_Texts/Lanciani/LANPAC/6*.html.

Leitner, Thomas K., and Ethan Romero-Severson, "Computer Simulations Predict the Spread of HIV," Los Alamos National Laboratory (August 1, 2018), https://discover.lanl.gov/news/0801-hiv-computer-simulations.

Licklider, J.C.R., "Man-Computer Symbiosis," *IRE Transactions on Human Factors in Electronics* vol. HFE-1 (March 1960), https://groups.csail.mit.edu/medg/people/psz/Licklider.html.

Linn, Andrew, Carole Khaw, Hugh Kildea, and Anne Tonkin, "Clinical Reasoning: A Guide to Improving Teaching and Practice," *Australian Family Physician* vol. 41, no. 1 (January–February 2012): 18–20, https://www.racgp.org.au/getattachment/5a28b3eb-5984-47f7-88a0-843e89537a4c/Clinical-reasoning.aspx.

Marchione, Marilynn, "Chinese Researcher Claims First Gene-Edited Babies," Associated Press (November 26, 2018), https://apnews.com

/ article / ap-top-news-international-news-ca-state-wire-genetic
-frontiers-health-4997bb7aa36c45449b488e19ac83e86d.

Markoff, John, "How Many Computers to Identify a Cat? 16,000," *The New York Times* (June 25, 2012), https://www.nytimes.com/2012/06/26 / technology / in-a-big-network-of-computers-evidence-of-machine -learning.html.

McAfee, "Chameleon: The Wi-Fi Virus That Hides in Plain Sight & Spreads Like a Cold," McAfee Blog (March 5, 2014), https://www.mcafee .com/blogs/privacy-identity-protection/chameleon-wifi-virus/.

Murray, Marjorie A., "Our Sense of Sight Part 1: Eye Anatomy and Function," https://faculty.washington.edu/chudler/eyetr.html.

Neubauer, Ian, "Top AIDS Researchers Killed in Malaysia Airlines Crash," *Time* (July 18, 2014), https://time.com/3003840/malaysia-airlines -ukraine-crash-top-aids-researchers-killed-aids2014-mh17/.

Norman, Dorothy, "Alfred Stieglitz—Seer," *Aperture* (1955), https://issues .aperture.org/article/1955/4/4/alfred-stieglitz-seer.

"Observe," Online Etymology Dictionary, https://www.etymonline.com / search?q=observe.

O'Gieblyn, Meghan, "Is the Internet Conscious? If It Were, How Would We Know?," *Wired* (September 16, 2020), https://www.wired.com/story / is-the-internet-conscious-if-it-were-how-would-we-know/.

O'Rourke, Meghan, "Finding a Metaphor for Your Loss," *Slate* (February 24, 2009), https://slate.com/human-interest/2009/02/the-long -goodbye-finding-a-metaphor-for-your-loss.html.

"Our Work," International Partnership for Microbicides (September 21, 2018), http://web.archive.org/web/20180921112920/https://www .ipmglobal.org/our-work.

Paulson, Steve, "The Nature of Consciousness: How the Internet Could Learn to Feel," *The Atlantic* (August 22, 2012), https://www.theatlantic .com/health/archive/2012/08/the-nature-of-consciousness-how-the -internet-could-learn-to-feel/261397/.

"Perception," Wikipedia, https://en.wikipedia.org/wiki/Perception.

Periyakoil, Vyjeyanthi S., "Using Metaphors in Medicine," *Journal of Palliative Medicine* vol. 11, no. 6 (January 15, 2008), https://www.liebertpub.com/doi/10.1089/jpm.2008.9885.

"Pneumocystis Pneumonia—Los Angeles," *Morbidity and Mortality Weekly Report* (June 5, 1981), https://www.cdc.gov/mmwr/preview/mmwrhtml/june_5.htm.

"Rabies," Wikipedia, https://en.wikipedia.org/wiki/Rabies.

Rapezzi, Claudio, Roberto Ferrari, and Angelo Branzi, "White Coats and Fingerprints: Diagnostic Reasoning in Medicine and Investigative Methods of Fictional Detectives," *British Medical Journal* vol. 331, no. 7531 (December 24, 2005), https://www.ncbi.nlm.nih.gov/pmc/articles/PMC1322237/.

Regalado, Antonio, "China's CRISPR Twins Might Have Had Their Brains Inadvertently Enhanced," *MIT Technology Review* (February 21, 2019), https://www.technologyreview.com/2019/02/21/137309/the-crispr-twins-had-their-brains-altered/.

"Seeing Is Believing," Reddit, https://www.reddit.com/r/todayilearned/comments/5dkq9e/til_the_oftenquoted_idiom_seeing_is_believing/.

"Sherlock Holmes and Dr. Joseph Bell," Conan Doyle Info (May 24, 2015), https://www.conandoyleinfo.com/sherlock-holmes/sherlock-holmes-and-dr-joseph-bell/.

Smothers, Hannah, "'Haunting' Is the Horrific New Dating Trend That's Even Worse Than Ghosting," *Cosmopolitan* (April 19, 2017), https://www.cosmopolitan.com/sex-love/a9524120/you-must-be-haunting-me/.

Sterling, Bruce, "Minitel: Cyberspace Sovereignty Decades Ago," *Wired* (June 21, 2017), https://www.wired.com/beyond-the-beyond/2017/06/minitel-cyberspace-sovereignty-decades-ago/.

Stock, Peter G., Burc Barin, Barbara Murphy, et al., "Outcomes of Kidney Transplantation in HIV-Infected Recipients," *The New England Journal of Medicine* vol. 363 (November 18, 2010), https://www.nejm.org /doi/full/10.1056/NEJMoa1001197.

Thibodeau, Paul H., and Lera Boroditsky, "Metaphors We Think With: The Role of Metaphor in Reasoning," *PLOS One* (February 23, 2011), https://journals.plos.org/plosone/article?id=10.1371/journal.pone .0016782.

Ulanoff, Lance, "Researchers Create Computer Virus That Spreads Like a Cold," *Mashable* (March 5, 2014), https://mashable.com/archive /chameleon-computer-virus.

"Update: Mortality Attributable to HIV Infection Among Persons Aged 25–44 Years—United States, 1991 and 1992," *Morbidity and Mortality Weekly Report* (November 19, 1993), https://www.cdc.gov/mmwr /preview/mmwrhtml/00022174.htm.

"Viral Phenomenon," Wikipedia, https://en.wikipedia.org/wiki/Viral _phenomenon.

"Viruses," Microbiology Society, https://microbiologysociety.org/why -microbiology-matters/what-is-microbiology/viruses.html.

Waddell, Kaveh, "The Computer Virus That Haunted Early AIDS Research-ers: The First-Ever Ransomware Attack Was Delivered on a Floppy Disk," *The Atlantic* (May 10, 2016), https://www.theatlantic.com/ technology/archive/2016/05/the-computer-virus-that-haunted -early-aids-researchers/481965/.

Winkler, Elizabeth, "The Viral Imagination," *Los Angeles Review of Books* (November 17, 2014), https://lareviewofbooks.org/article/viral -imagination/.

"World's First Gene-Edited Babies Created in China, Claims Scientist," *The Guardian* (November 26, 2018), https://www.theguardian.com /science/2018/nov/26/worlds-first-gene-edited-babies-created-in -china-claims-scientist.

Zimmer, Carl, "Sizing Up Consciousness by Its Bits," *The New York Times* (September 20, 2010), https://www.nytimes.com/2010/09/21/science/21consciousness.html.

Zittrain, Jonathan, "A History of IP in 50 Objects: Internet," (June 2019), https://cyber.harvard.edu/sites/default/files/2019-06/2019-06_zittrainIP.pdf.

———, "The Internet Is Rotting," *The Atlantic* (June 30, 2021), https://www.theatlantic.com/technology/archive/2021/06/the-internet-is-a-collective-hallucination/619320/.

TV AND FILM

Arnold, Andrea, dir., *Transparent*. Season 2, episode 10, "Grey Green Brown & Copper." Aired February 1, 2016, on Amazon Prime Video.

Fryman, Pamela, dir., *Frasier*. Season 6, episode 24, "Shutout in Seattle: Part 2." Aired May 20, 1999, on NBC.

Fukunaga, Cary Joji, dir., *True Detective*. Season 1, episode 3, "The Locked Room." Aired January 26, 2014, on HBO.

Hardy, Rod, dir., *Battlestar Galactica*. Season 2, episode 5, "The Farm." Aired August 12, 2005, on the Sci-Fi Channel.

Paterson, Nigel, and Ben J. Wilson, dirs., *The Beginning and End of the Universe*. Aired March 22–29, 2016, on BBC Four.

Sackheim, Daniel, dir., *True Detective*. Season 3, episode 8, "Now Am Found." Aired February 4, 2019, on HBO.

Schlamme, Thomas, dir., *The West Wing*. Season 2, episode 10, "Noël." Aired December 13, 2000, on NBC.

The Wachowskis, dirs., *The Matrix*. Burbank, Calif.: Warner Bros. Pictures, 1999.

Whitmore, James, Jr., dir., *The Good Wife*. Season 1, episode 23, "Running." Aired May 25, 2010, on CBS.

PODCASTS AND RADIO

"Antibodies Part 1: CRISPR," *Radiolab* (June 6, 2015).

"Black Box," *Radiolab* (January 17, 2014).

"Patient Zero," *Radiolab* (November 15, 2011).

"The French Connection," *Reply All* (January 17, 2015).

"One Last Thing Before I Go," *This American Life* (September 23, 2016).

ABOUT THE AUTHOR

HEATHER MCCALDEN is a multidisciplinary artist working with text, image, and movement. A graduate of the Royal College of Art, she has been awarded residencies by the Banff Centre for Arts and Creativity and Mahler & LeWitt Studios. *The Observable Universe,* winner of the Fitzcarraldo Editions/ Mahler & LeWitt Studios Essay Prize, is her first book. She lives in New York City.

ABOUT THE TYPE

This book was set in Dante, a typeface designed by Giovanni Mardersteig (1892–1977). Conceived as a private type for the Officina Bodoni in Verona, Italy, Dante was originally cut only for hand composition by Charles Malin, the famous Parisian punch cutter, between 1946 and 1952. Its first use was in an edition of Boccaccio's *Trattatello in laude di Dante* that appeared in 1954. The Monotype Corporation's version of Dante followed in 1957. Though modeled on the Aldine type used for Pietro Cardinal Bembo's treatise *De Aetna* in 1495, Dante is a thoroughly modern interpretation of that venerable face.

NOTE ABOUT THE TEXT

This book was written over a six-year period beginning in 2016 and ending in 2021. During this time many of the referenced URLs, web articles, and Wikipedia pages have either transformed entirely or no longer exist. In a sense the book suffers from link rot, in what is perhaps the first case of a digital malady affecting a material object. Of course, some of the physical locations and businesses mentioned have also disappeared, all of which is to say: the text you are reading is already a souvenir.